# PHA
# RMA
# KON

'In all things there is a poison, and there is nothing without a poison. It depends only upon the dose whether a poison is a poison or not.'

Paracelsus

*This one goes out to the one I Love*

For Helen

- without whom this book would never have been written.

'nothing is true, everything is permitted'

attributed to Hassan-i Sabbah

Naturally though this book discusses all sorts of things that are currently illegal in many nations I would never wish to encourage anyone to break the Law. Moreover since this book contains information about how human beings can fly like birds, become transformed into animals and explore the farthest reaches of inner space it is, quite clearly, a work of fiction.

# PHARMAKON

Drugs and the Imagination

## Julian Vayne

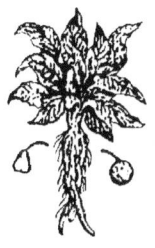

Copyright © 2006 Mandrake & Liminalspace Publications

First print edition

**First e-book edition 2001 El-cheapo Books
ISBN 1-903548-11-4**

All rights reserved. No part of this work may be reproduced or utilized in any form by any means electronic or mechanical, including *xerography, photocopying, microfilm*, and *recording*, or by any information storage system without permission in writing from the publishers.

Also available
Now That's What I Call Chaos Magick (with Greg Humphries)

Seeds of Magick
Personal Development with the Tarot
The Inner Space Workbook
(all above titles Julian Vayne with Catherine Summers)

Published by
Mandrake of Oxford
PO Box 250
OXFORD
OX1 1AP (UK)

A CIP catalogue record for this book is available from the British Library and the US Library of Congress.

**1869928741**

# Contents

Thank You ................................................................................. 7

Second Time Around –
Preface to the Second Edition ............................................... 9

Intro ........................................................................................ 12

Essence – defining drug experience .................................... 22

Shamania – the secret history of drugs .............................. 44

Perfect Mystery – drugs, the mind and the human brain ................. 67

Odditorium – the dual process of the mind ....................... 87

Movements of a Visionary – drugs and the occult ........... 132

Blood, Sugar, Sex, Magick – drugs in esoteric culture ................. 145

Break on Through – the experience of drugs ................... 177

The Modern Things - drugs, transgression and society ................. 221

Notes ..................................................................................... 237

Bibliography ........................................................................ 269

Index ..................................................................................... 275

JULIAN VAYNE

# Thank You

This book represents the confluence of a number of ideas, experiences and, most importantly, the shared wisdom of some of my best friends.

Thanks to Eddie Marcus for being an inspiration, a constant source of new ideas and argument in the best sense of the word. Thanks also to Richard Sutcliffe, Leah Watkins, Paul Harris, Tariq Edwards, Dave Cartwright, Steve Robinson (especially for his introduction to the work of Derrida), Holly Hammond and Steven 'Rocky' Rockcliffe for their companionship, ideas and insight. I'd like to extend thanks to my medical mates who, apart from being cool and groovy people, have also fed me some excellent expertise from their disciplines (special thanks to Alexa for her comments on the 'neurobollocks' section). My love and thanks go out to Professor Ronald Hutton for his help, support and friendship and to Alex for helping me close this particular chapter in my life by introducing me to Dimitri.

There are many other friends who have supported and assisted me during the three or so years that I've been thinking about writing this book; Dr

Christopher Kemp, Rose, Dan, Sara, Mark, Ali, Su, Charlie, Tsubi and Lou (cheers for the proofing), The Montpelier Massive (York and Richmond Chapters) and many others - love and blessings to you all.

And finally; thank you to all those good people who regularly contribute to the growing drug related resources on the internet – you know who you are.

J.

# Second Time Around :
# Preface to the Second Edition

It's curious looking back on one's work. My words on the page are both immediately familiar and yet curiously disconnected from the me of now. When I was offered the opportunity to re-issue Pharmakon (the first edition having been a limited, small run publication) I was considered the possibility of a full re-write. Looking back at the text there are certainly some things that might be amended. However, with a few corrections and the addition of an index and full bibliography, I've let the original text stand unchanged. Pharmakon is the book I wrote then in 2001, in a sense this was my self-imposed doctoral thesis (I've always liked to claim the title doctor, though I'll admit immediately that I'm only a doctor in the sense that the palmist at the end of the pier is a professor). The quasi-academic style of writing is quite different to the more autobiographical material of *Now That's What I Call Chaos Magick*. If I had decided to re-write this book I'd probably be placing more emphasis on Internet sources. The wonderful on-line library of drug information Erowid (to which some of the profit from this volume will be donated) would be an even more key source that it was for me in 2001. Other areas of the net, including the proliferation of sites retailing the latest consciousness changing agents, have also grown substantially since the first publication of Pharmakon.

Other developments, such as the Exploring Consciousness conference in Bath, England and, as I write, the planned LSD conference in Switzerland (to celebrate the 100th birthday of Albert Hofmann) have unfolded. On a personal level I have been able to continue some of the personal explorations of materials described I this book, although today my main attention is on exploring consciousness not through drugs but through the experience of raising my children.

Pharmakon barely touches the legal issues surrounding drug use. Indeed this was a deliberate policy (as I make clear in the book) because the situation is one that requires a volume all of it's own. As I write this a friend and fellow magician is incarcerated at Her Majesty's pleasure for possession of various controlled substances. The British government is being pulled both ways by an intelligent program of decriminalisation for cannabis and the reactionary desire to enact harsher penalties for possession and use of other drugs. Meanwhile the mainstream media presents us with the fearful spectre of binge drinking on the one hand, while licensing legislation is being radically revised to increase the availability of alcohol on the other. Our culture is caught in an insane doublethink that, I dearly hope, we can begin to transform. To this end I am more and more aware that Pagans should be one of the groups who are standing up for cognitive freedom and the traditional right to use 'plant allies' to explore the universe.

The thing that stands in our way is, of course, fear. Fear of drug addiction, fear of violent crime born out of that addiction, fear of madness, illness, and death resulting from the use of drugs. This fear is certainly part of the real experience of drugs, if nothing else (although I might use slightly different language now) my use of the term transgression denotes this. Once you've taken that hit of LSD there isn't any kind of safe word, you're in for a trip and the only way to overcome fear is to give up, to give in, to ride the snake. It is, I believe, this fear of giving in that leads to our culture of fear and repressive (and ineffective) legislation around drugs. What we fear is the abyss of losing control, but as any Master or Mistress of the temple will tell you, it's only by giving ourselves up to the abyss that we can come to real understanding of who we are.

Enjoy this book, stay high and stay free.

Julian Vayne, Devon 2005

# Intro

## History

The analysis of drugs presented here is framed within the context of a number of different areas of study; ethnography, neurochemistry, literature and others. But the underlying language throughout this book is that of modern occultism. Occultism is the study of 'that which is hidden'. In practice this tends to mean areas of human experience which could be glossed as being the parapsychological or mystical. The exact definition of what constitutes 'the occult' is wide open to question. For some people it means the use of tarot cards, for others complex Neo-Pagan belief systems, for some the study of paranormal or anomalous phenomena (such as ghosts, UFOs or syncronicity). In the context of this book occultism can be broadly considered to be *the study and practice of engaging with mystery.*

The exploration and realisation of our hidden (occult) selves, through a variety of different techniques is what I mean by occultism. To appreciate our 'occult self' is to examine all that is hidden, repressed or excluded by our exoteric (outward) being. In practice this means employing the methods of people who, in modern culture, have been called mystics, visionaries, shamans, magicians. But this does not mean scientists, artists or engineers cannot or do not explore the occult, and we will meet many people in our story who are proof of this.

One important means of exploring our 'occult selves' is drug experience, and this is the focus of this book. The many different and diverse aspects of drug exploration are a fascinating lens through which to view the practice of occultism (or 'magic') in action.

## Safety Dance

A Word of Warning - I have tried to ensure that the information, especially any 'practical comments' about drugs and drug use are accurate. However this book is not intended to be a trippers' manual. Most of the information here I have checked as thoroughly as I can. However an error on my part here, a glitch in the printing press there, and problems can arise. People who are involved in using drugs for 'self exploration' (for lack of a better term), and most of those who use drugs recreationally, are very sensible. But when the drug is one you haven't tried before, or if you are uncertain about issues such 'can I drink alcohol if I've taken MDMA?' or 'what is the usual dose of 2-CB?' – check your facts! Find at least two sources of information and check things out, find somebody whose opinion you trust and ask them – just to be on the safe side.

## Summoning of the Muse.

Drugs straddle a boundary. They exist as physical substances, as social constructs, as the generators of experiences and even as economic entities in a shadowy 'liminal state' - that is the threshold realm 'between worlds'.[1] Taken as a whole the world of 'drugs' comprises the legal and illegal. Substances that are natural and others that are artificial. They can provide us with access to states that verge on heaven or may seem like hell.

Taking drugs can be a magical act. When I refer to 'magic' I am talking about the desire, the individual 'project' to deliberately enter into this liminal space. The desire to commune with 'the other' is 'magical desire'. (The other being simply all that we do not, generally, recognise as being 'self'. It is the *mystery* in my definition of occultism).

The magical use of drugs - the use of drugs to enter the 'liminal state' has echoes in many classically 'occult' areas of study. An example of this may be found within alchemy.

Alchemy represented a form of science which included what we might call a 'spiritual dimension' and a perception of the whole universe as being 'alive'. For the alchemists of yore there was no division between living things and dead matter, nor between matter and mind. For them, I suspect, the idea that you could use an extract of the lowly cannabis weed to see God would not have seemed strange at all.

For the ancient alchemists there were two fundamental processes continuously active in the universe: *solve* (dissolving/analysis) and *coagula* (recombining/synthesising). A variety of alchemical (or 'occult') techniques sought to create a 'universal solvent' (or 'philosophers stone') which could dissolve the leaden world and reconstitute it into the gold of spiritual illumination. Drugs, existing as I hope to show they do, in the liminal state (that is, between the worlds of matter and mind, spirit and substance), can be just such a Philosopher's Stone; materials capable of transforming the universe, of conferring new insights and abilities.

Magical use of drugs echoes alchemy in another sense, in that the 'lowest' stuff, the thing that can itself lead to our downfall, is used in the 'highest' or most noble pursuit. It is from 'base lead' that we can forge the brilliant gold of ecstatic or 'numinous' experience.

My own interest in drugs comes from my background as a practising occultist. I have spent some years using techniques such as the tarot, ritual drama, sex and meditative practices to explore the occult other. Over the course of the last five years I have been employing the use of drugs as another magical technique.

On a personal level I have found exploring drugs to be a truly transformative, at times harrowing, but frequently illuminating process. For me this book, and the experiences that have lead to its production, have been a personal alchemy. I wouldn't necessarily say that what I have learnt from my studies has made me a better person (though I hope that it has). But I am certain that through drugs I have been fortunate to have experienced a powerful method of engaging with 'the other', and transforming and exploring my sense of self. I would certainly say that many of the experiences I have had over the last five years have, without doubt, been some of the most powerful ones I have ever encountered as an adult.

The grandfather of modern hallucinogenic pharmacology, Alexander Shulgin echoes my own intense feelings about drug experience when he recounts his first psychedelic journey with mescaline. 'It was a day that will remain blazingly clear in my memory…I understood that our entire universe is contained in the mind and the spirit. We may not choose to find access to it, we may even deny its existence, but it is indeed there inside us, and there are chemicals that can catalyse its availability.'[2]

Such a breakthrough in understanding, of the type that Shulgin gained through mescaline, arises from the process that I refer to as 'transgression'. Transgression is a complex concept which resists a limited definition in just the same way as the Chinese mystical concept of the *tao* does. Therefore throughout this book I use slightly different terms for the transgressive process, slightly different analogies and models. The aim here is not to confuse the reader but instead to explore these ideas from many different viewpoints.

But for now, as a working definition, let me say that *transgression is the process whereby the individual crosses the liminal space between Self and Other*. Let me attempt to make things clearer by stating at the outset what transgression is not.

The transgressive experience that I talk about is explicitly 'of the world'. This isn't an aesthetic, turning away from 'the world, the flesh and the devil' and retreating into an abstracted 'other worldly' mystical paradise. Like the transformations of alchemy, the occult use of drugs is firmly rooted in the world of matter and the body. The occult philosophies that I am most interested in do not imagine the world as a veil of sorrows or suffering. Nor do they see the goal of self-knowledge to be the transcendence of the earthly realm, and the rejection of the 'base' in favour of some kind of disembodied higher state. Magic (in the modern sense) seeks to directly engage with the world, and to experience the existence of spirit embodied in matter, and matter arising out of spirit.

In the case of physical drugs the material realm itself serves as our lever of liberation. Moreover the drug taker can return to the world, bringing with her a reformed sense of self. The self of the drug taker is changed, but remains a 'self'. The obliteration of individual consciousness isn't the goal - instead the aim is transformation, re-formulation and reintegration of the Self. The Self is liberated by, through, and in the world. We are not talking here about turning our backs on either nature or culture, nor of blandly privileging one over the other. As Albert Hofmann, the discoverer of LSD puts it in '*LSD My Problem Child*';

> 'We are not leading up to a sentimental enthusiasm for nature, to "back to nature" in Rousseau's sense. That Romantic Movement, which sought the idyll in nature, can also be explained by a feeling of humankind's separation from nature. What is needed today is a fundamental re-experience of the oneness of all living things, a comprehensive reality consciousness that ever more infrequently develops spontaneously, the more the primordial flora and fauna of our mother earth must yield to a dead technological environment.'[3]

The occult use of drugs, by the very fact that drugs are physical materials, affirms the 'oneness' that Hofmann speaks of. It collapses the dividing lines of Self and Other through the process of transgression. The apparently opposite, separate qualities of matter and mind, nature and culture, subject and object are destabilised. And, as Hofmann remarks, this process may be a very good thing for modern society.

Drug experience isn't Romantic (in the historical sense of the term). Transgression, whether through drugs or not, does not seek to turn our feet to a better path because we are lost in the domain of culture. We only think that we need to get back to Eden because we consider ourselves 'fallen'. Trangressive experience can fracture such myths of division, calling them into question and nibbling away at their borders.

Neither is the process of transgression anti-rational, anti-logical. It does not strive towards the obliteration of consciousness nor intelligence. Taking drugs for 'magical purposes' is a rational desire. Our drive to engage with the magical nature of drugs emerges, in part, out of our individual intellect.

Although, given the state of contemporary western society, this book may at times dwell on the notion of going 'beyond the rational approach', of reductionist materialism or contemporary science, I am not at all opposed to logical, abstract and intellectual thought. I believe that by exploring the magical power of drugs to transform the Self we can have our cake and eat it. As the alchemical conception of the universe includes both processes (the analysis of logical/sequential/artificial thought and the synthesis of irrational/holistic/natural emotions), so transgression partakes of those domains we usually think of as separate (emotional and rational).

So transgression does not mean leaving behind our humanity and propelling ourselves into the idealised world of the noble savage or childlike innocence. Nor does it mean that one must be 'living on the edge' in the glamorised madness of the post-modern period. As Alan W Watts[4] points out '...we do not need to abandon culture and return to some precivilized level, for neither in the drug experience nor in more general forms of mystical experience does one lose the skills or the knowledge which civilization has produced.'

Instead this occult investigation, this sacred transgression through drugs, can mean exploring the active ability (the *magical ability*) to play between the poles of duality, to collapse the divides of subject and object and to re-emerge into a new sense of being. A form of being that can permit the existence of dualism and paradox, of distinctions such as nature and culture but can simultaneously seek to destabilise, fracture and unite into new configurations these categories as part of the ongoing process of becoming who we can be.

## Explain Myself

There are a few additional points that I would ask the reader to note before we begin our story.

In the second section of this book I have used much of the language of science. However this is not because I want to ground my thesis in a scientifically authoritative manner. If nothing else the field of neurochemistry is so complex[5] and evolving so fast that what is accepted hard science today is just as likely to be overturned tomorrow. Rather, contemporary neurological theory can provide another set of symbols, another story, through which we can explore the relationship of drugs and the human psyche. Although I am interested in the neurochemical effects of drugs I believe that it is an impoverished view of drug experience that does not include the psyche as well as the body.

As I have said my primary interest is occultism. For me drug experience is one expression of the techniques of producing altered states of awareness that magic is all about. The vocabulary of modern occultism (the field of study that generally lays claim to the word 'magic'[6]) is very specialised. Most of the writers that have influenced my own work are modern occultists. Their work tends to appear in journals or in short run, or privately published books. I have tried to keep my use of esoteric language to a minimum in this book though it is really very much about occultism – the phenomena of drug experience as an entry (transgression) into the liminal world is my vehicle, but my central subject is magic.

Defining what magic is is virtually impossible; it is a slippery term precisely because it deals with the intentional act of entering the liminal, transformative realm.[7] So, by examining drugs I am actually examining the concept of magic, albeit indirectly.

Most of the time when I use the word 'drug' within these pages I am referring to a broad class of materials that are capable of changing consciousness, of affecting the mind and the sense of Self. In general, when I use the term 'drug experience' I mean an experience which may provide access to a numinous experience, a 'peak moment' or at least a shift in awareness of, and changes in the construction of, ones sense of 'I'.[8] A drug experience in these terms means a moment when the boundary between Self and Other is, if not shattered, then at least relaxed and rendered permeable.

Most of the drugs that I examine in detail in this book are what are usually called hallucinogens (I will return to what this term means exactly later). However I certainly do not preclude the possibility that the process of magical transformation (entering the liminal space) can be accomplished with other drugs - e.g. cocaine, heroin, alcohol, etc. Indeed even those chemicals that seem to provide so little effect in the habitual user (such as tobacco) can, under the right conditions become agents of transformation. In fact in some respects this is one of the most vital points to remember when reading this book. Drugs are materials that can, quite literally, change your mind, and as I shall show what we decide to call a drug is a moot point. For most of us the transcendent power in the thunderclouds, in the smell of the soil or the cry of orgasm is, if not actively oppressed then is, at least generally, suppressed. The entire world tends towards the transcendent, the transformative and the magical (human nature doubly so).[9] What we generally recognise as 'drugs' and particularly 'hallucinogenic drugs' are particularly potent zones of transformative power at this point in our history. As such they are potent keys to our transformation of being, into whatever it is we shall and can become.

Of course drug use (as we generally understand the term) is a powerful way to explore the relationship of Self and Other, but it is by no means the only way.

# Essence:
# defining drug experience

### Adrift on Deep Water

The boundary of any concept is hazy. Although, as human beings, we spend a lot of time categorising the world. The definition of any category, any exact meaning, becomes more elusive the more we search for it. Try it yourself – we all know the difference between a mug and a cup but where does that difference lie?

In discussing definitions of, and the meaning of drug experience in particular we have to remember some important principles. These are philosophical ideas that I feel must underpin our analysis of drug experience. They represent important insights into the way we describe the world and have huge implications for very specific questions such as 'what does such-and-such a drug do to the human mind?'

- Language (spoken, written, signed etc.) exists as a network of relationships. These relationships are formed by *differences*. The word 'pig' means what it does because of what it is not (e.g. 'fig', 'dog', 'god' etc.) This type of categorisation of relationships was the focus of the structuralist movement in philosophy and writers such as Saussure. According to post-modern philosophy the structuralist relationships of language are produced and maintained by *Power*. That is the interaction of different stories or *discourses* which seek to define themselves (very often) by what they are not, by self created, relative (rather than 'objective' or 'absolute') notions of difference.

- That all concepts contain not only their opposite (in the dualistic way that black implies white and height necessitates depth), but that a category that apparently exists only by exclusion of something, also contains that very something at its heart. This idea is called 'the trace' from the 'deconstruction' of the philosopher Derrida who suggests that words do not simply exist as networks of exclusions but also that words *imply* each other through difference. For instance the word 'pig' contains certain sounds – p-i-g. The sound 'p' is not only the difference, the exclusion of the other sounds in the language but also *exists by virtue of them*. This is like the drawing exercise where, rather than drawing the tree, the art student draws the spaces around the tree, and this *allows* the shape of the tree to *emerge* on the page.

When we come to examine what a drug actually is, it is important to remember these two points. Rather than talk about 'drugs' we are often better off looking at the relationship of drugs to other concepts (for example, drug vs. food) and who has the power to maintain these differences and why.

We can also look for Derridas' 'trace' in drugs. We can examine paradoxical effects in which the drug does quite the reverse of what we would usually expect. We can also examine the way that a drug experience is defined, as much by what is around it as by the action of the chemical itself.

So from structuralism we can remember to ask – what is the difference being proposed between one 'drug' and another?

From post-modernism we can ask – what discourse, what stories are told about drugs and why?

From deconstruction (or post-structuralism) we can ask – what are the paradoxes, where is the 'play', the sliding around of what drugs *mean* and what they are supposed to *do*?

## Chemistry

Any substance that changes the chemistry of the body might be said to be a drug. (Commentators are usually quick to point out that we often implicitly limit the use of the term 'drug' to medical or illicit substances).[10] If we assume, just for the moment, that the mind is a system based on a chemical network (the brain and body) then anything that we come into contact with might be thought of as a drug; since each experience might be considered to be 'chemical' in nature (including our sense of Self). So it is understandable that the experience of falling in love is often equated with a drug induced intoxication. To take another example; being startled by a thunderclap can massively change the chemical state of the body, but is the thunderclap a drug?

If we imagine that our minds are related to, and also emerge from, the neurochemical network of our bodies we cannot help but assume that, in a broad sense, all modes of experience are drug states. The snarl of the dog that raises the pulse or the cooing of an infant that stimulates lactation are, in this broad sense, chemical experiences. Although we are admittedly using a wide definition of 'drug' here the point is that the boundary of the word can be extended this far and it is important to remember this. As we get closer to the 'substance' of the chemical effect it is easy to forget that the boundaries of the drug experience can and do include social and environmental factors.

Even with more immediate physical substances that can be ingested, the blurring of definitions continues. A hot chilli will make you sweat, increase your heart rate and may even lead to addictive behaviours but we would rarely consider chilli a drug. On the other hand, if you swallow chalk tablets, having been first convinced they are mild MDMA, you may well feel a rush of energy, some measure of empathic feeling with others and quite possibly become 'intoxicated'. Certainly there has been a chemical alteration of the body but is a placebo itself a drug?

Drug experiences can be tremendously diverse. The experienced effect of one physical material, of a known dosage, even on the same person, can be widely different on different occasions. Depending on the situation any drug may also have 'paradoxical effects'. Amphetamine, for instance, is used therapeutically to calm hyperactivity in children,[11] but can make other individuals sleepy or, more usually, intensely active.[12]

To throw the boundary of drug/not drug into more confusion, in the modern period we are getting used to the idea of 'mood altering' drugs that make their user 'normal' (for example the much vaunted serotonin modifier Prozac). We should not think that the idea of using drugs to change moods is a new phenomenon. In Medieval writings a drug that worked on the 'bile humour' was as much effecting a physical as an emotional and even moral aspect of the patient's person. We also have examples of drugs used in complementary therapy, such as Bach flower remedies. So although we might be familiar with, say, pine for clearing a blocked nose, as a Bach remedy it is for those '...who blame themselves, even for the mistakes of others,' and who suffer from feelings of 'self-reproach even when they have done no wrong.'[13]

Today we live in an age when what were previously thought to be social or spiritual conditions (e.g. love, depression or madness) may be seen in terms of brain chemistry. We live in an age when 'normal' functioning of your body and mind might be supported by the use of drugs (aspirin for heart trouble, Viagra for impotence, seretonin reuptake inhibitors for unhappiness).

# Drugs

So what of opium, cocaine, acid - the things we all know to be drugs? These materials are ones that we can ingest that will certainly change our chemistry. There is a lot to be learnt from looking at and examining the chemical action of drugs. Both in highly abstract ways (such as producing a computer model to show how MDMA effects serotonin reuptake in a brain), and in terms of observable behaviours and personal accounts. The materials that we commonly call drugs are the instigators of a particular set of processes. These processes are so profound that they can radically change the functions of the person to whom they are administered.

But before we begin to look at the effects of drugs we must shrug off the old idea that we have a 'normal' or 'straight' self upon which a drug exerts its' effects. If being depressed is not normal, but Prozac makes one happier where do we locate the normal sense of self? Post-modern writers might tend to locate this 'normal self' in the discourses of society as a whole – depression is not 'normal' because society (or rather the discourses of medicine, economics, the family etc. that are dominant in our society, say that depression is not normal) deems it so. But the notion of normality is even more tenuous than the post-modern reading suggests. We have all had the experience of suddenly, perhaps upon waking one morning, feeling unexpectedly elated (that 'Christmas Eve feeling' is how one friend describes it). Or of unaccountable sadness without rhyme or reason. One might fall in love and experience all kinds of 'deviations' from one's 'normal' self. Indeed a rich diversity, even a certain degree of extremes of mental state (grief, elation) might be considered a prerequisite for a normal mentality.

In short, 'normal' has meaning in the sense that it is the average or most common state of being over a given period. But we must not confuse the idea of a usual state (normality) with ideas of general sanity, health or moral rectitude. On the one hand it may be 'normal' for a person to drink alcohol heavily each day if they are an alcoholic but we would rarely say this is healthy. Equally to have ingested 100 micrograms of LSD may make you feel anything but 'normal' though the desire to do so (perhaps as part of therapy to cure ones alcohol addition) may be far from pathological.

When we examine drug experience we should not place drug experience as the polar opposite of our normal 'straight' state. If one takes a drug one's normality has not been removed. To use Derrida's term,[14] the drug has supplemented (or complemented) one's normality.

To recapitulate; anything might be thought of as a drug. A potent drug is one that can so change our chemistry as to place us outside of the 'normal' patterns of human relationships. But where we put the boundaries of this 'normality' are open to question.

## Material World.

Most writers on art have their favourite artists. So too most writers on drugs have their favourite drugs. This is perfectly acceptable and understandable - I'll start off openly and say that mine are LSD and, in second place, MDMA. The problem is that those writers who feel that humans could learn from drug experiences frequently confuse personal preference with a general prescription. This is the classic trap that they should be more aware of since they tend to see one of the problems of modern society as being an obsession with materialism and products, rather than inner spiritual awareness.

The search to find a reliable tree of knowledge, a drug that would spiritually awaken humans on a consistant basis, has been on for at least 100 years. Since the death of god declared by Nietzsche (and others), we have had wave after wave of chemical prophets who have wanted to tell us exactly what humans are going to need to snort or toke before we can become 'Supermen'.

Aldous Huxley waxes lyrical about mescaline, while Timothy Leary extols LSD as the saviour chemical. Most recently Terrence McKenna has argued that it is tryptamine-based hallucinogens that will save us all. Some writers have projected with own favourite drug back into history. A classic example of this is to be found in the work of Wasson.[15] A ethnomycologist who, in attempting to discover the basis of the Hindu mystical material 'soma', became more and more fixated on the idea that fly agaric was the answer.

To be fair many writers on drugs, including those mentioned above (in most instances), do attempt to place their favourite chemical in a broader context. Few drug writers over the last 50 years have failed to point out that just sniffing a line of miracle chemical X is unlikely to have the effect of turning everyone into a 'groovy person'. However there is still a general tendency to imagine that there is one key drug, one saviour chemical. This desire for a, literal, wonder drug, is totally understandable in the context of western mass-produced society. If we are going to have an answer to life, the universe and everything, its got to be one answer. One creed, one grand unified theory of everything, and one chemical gnosis.

Drugs can have different effects depending on a literally infinite number of factors (from what you had to eat, to the last film you saw, to the fact that your trip is undertaken close to the ocean).[16] What I believe is important is not the drug so much as the *drug experience*. Moreover it is not simply a question of taking drugs to partake fully of the experience but neither is it necessarily a question of elaborate formalised ceremony and training.

## Saviour Machine

As well as using drugs, there are many other ways of entering the liminal realm. In terms of drug use some writers prefer to emphasise the drug (the 'saviour chemical'), whereas others stress the preparation of the mind and body prior to the attempt. Huxley, during his experiments with mescaline, came to believe that the lengthy ritual preparation for the use of hallucinogens was largely unnecessary. Equally Leary believed (at least in his earlier writings) that, although 'set and setting'[17] were important, there was no need for elaborate preparation before taking LSD. Again these beliefs are symptomatic of a product based view of the world, where drugs are external stuff that we take and have definable effects.

In ancient religion, according to writers such as Wasson, the mystical crux of ceremony was taking the holy drug. Indeed the very root of religion and the emergence of human consciousness itself might well be the result of a specific drug (*amanita muscaria* in the work of Wasson, *psilocybe* in the writings of McKenna). Once again the complex network of relationships which defines what a drug is are submerged in the monolithic idea that a particular chemical is *the* answer. This emphasis plays down the complexity of the spiritual or religious impulse in humanity. A drug (the wine of the mass, the peyote of native American religion) may be a focal and important part of a spiritual tradition but it is not the *raison d'être* for human spirituality. Rather spirituality is the context within which the drug is taken, and in terms of which the experience of intoxication is interpreted.

We do have plenty of ancient historical texts that describe divine intoxication. Many of these intoxications are referred to in terms of religious ecstatic experience and may well have been linked to the use of drugs. But we must also appreciate that, just as drugs might catalyse religious insight, so too drug experience can be used as a metaphor or description of mystical spontaneous mystical illumination. In ancient western religion we know that the use of alcohol was widespread and there may well have been other drugs employed. For instance in the classical rites of Eleusis it has been conjectured that ergot (which contains LSD like alkaloids) was used, though this is unlikely since a common effect of repeated ergot intoxication is gangrene. Historians and ethnobotonists have proposed other candidates for the Eleusis drug including McKenna's suggestion of psilocybe mushrooms.

Intoxication often features in mythology. For example in Hinduism where lord Shiva sits up in the Himalayas, smoking dope all day. But it is primarily from the Americas that we have the best documented and contemporary knowledge concerning the use of drugs in a 'traditional spiritual' context. Yet even within such 'psychedelic' societies drug use is not necessarily the centre of either these cultures as a whole, or what we might recognise as their spiritual practice in particular.

There are many ancient cultures and groups who may have used transformative drugs, though the emphasis is placed on the transformation, the magical experience itself, rather than on the drug. This might be because the knowledge of these herbs was itself sacred and secret. It may also be because the drug is the doorway but not itself the journey. In our culture we tend to look for the *reason*, the herb that is *responsible* for the mystical experience. This overlooks the fact that the drug experience occurs within a certain set and setting (e.g. the ceremonies of the Eleusis cult or the rituals of the native American peoples). As stated above the point is the transformative drug *experience*, not the drug material alone.

My own view is that, to be genuinely useful, drug experience needs to be of a certain type in order to be really transformative. We each have a context within which we place our drug experiences. Huxley is perhaps the best example of a writer who, after experimenting with mescaline, was able to contextualise his insights in the form of books. Huxley was already a writer when he took mescaline, but his writing certainly takes on a new dimension afterwards. In order to have a transformative drug experience it is necessary to have an internal system that can conceptualise, analyse and subject itself again to, the drug experience. So a religious belief that, say, LSD is a sacramental substance is only a transformative belief if it allows the believer to incorporate, analyse and return to the LSD experience remaining open to new insights. This process of understanding, considering, and re-engaging with the drug experience is the process of *learning*. The idea that the drug experience is itself both representative of and, in some ways, identical to the process of learning is a vitally important one. This process, this transformative engagement with the drug experience, and being able to use that experience to learn, is what I mean by using a drug as an act of transgression. To support this practice with techniques (such as ceremony, myth, or certain attitudes) is the practice of magic.

The magical use of drugs may come as a spontaneous knowledge. It may also be the result of training, either with drugs themselves or by using other methods of self-development and change. Any process can be carried out in a 'magical manner' - examples across time and culture include martial arts, ritual drama, sex, surfing, or meditative practice. As with many things in life - and with the magical use of drugs in particular - it ain't what you do, it's the way that you do it.

## Eat the Menu

There are any number of ways in which drugs may be classified. Perhaps the most commonly used system, in day-to-day use as well as (hidden within more complex terminology) in pharmacology, is a 'common sense' tripartite division;

*Downers* – drugs that make you relaxed, disconnected from 'reality', sleepy etc. e.g. opium.

*Uppers* – drugs that stimulate and excite, making the users feel engaged and alert. e.g. amphetamine.

*Psychedelics* – drugs that make the world seem weird. e.g. LSD.

A more formal system is used by Albert Hofmann, who, developing an older system of classification, recognises four broad categories:

*Analgesics and euphorics*. e.g. opium and coca.

*Sedatives*. e.g. reserpine

*Hypnotics*. e.g. kava kava

*Hallucinogens or psychotomimetics*. e.g. peyote, marihuana.[18]

The problem with even this simple and conventional classification is that the lines are not just blurred but often obliterated as the effect of one drug, and also of the same drug taken in different circumstances, can vary tremendously. For instance, MDMA is a modified amphetamine (chemically), but is gently psychedelic (in that it breaks down interpersonal boundaries) in it's action. It can act like an opiate in that it kills pain. Whereas an analgesic, such as ketamine, can produce hallucinations and, if taken over a long period, may begin to act more like a powerful amphetamine.

The 'classic' way of categorising drugs is that of Louis Lewin, one of the most important toxicologists of his time, who set forth his classification of drugs in *Phantastica* first published in 1924.

*Euphorica* – sedatives of mental activity, these substances diminish or even suspend the functions of emotion and perception

*Phantastica* – hallucinating substances

*Inebriantia* – causing cerebral excitation followed by depression.

*Hypnotica* – sleep producing agents

*Excitantia* – mental stimulants.

There are, of course, other ways of categorising drugs. Some systems of classification may seem 'unscientific' (and therefore less 'reasonable') but in reality they are all arbitrary or at least based on certain assumptions about what is significant and what is not.[19] In *777 & Other Qabalistic*

*Writings*, by occultist Aleister Crowley, drugs are classed with respect to a series of forces that are drawn from the 'Tree of Life' (the Qabalah) and in turn linked to astrological symbols:[20]

| Qabalistic Sephira | Astrological Symbol | Vegetable drugs |
|---|---|---|
| Kether | Pluto | Elixir Vitae |
| Chockmah | Neptune | Hashish |
| Binah | Saturn | Belladona |
| Chesed | Jupiter | Opium |
| Geburah | Mars | Tobacco, Nux Vomica, Nettle |
| Tipherath | Sun | Stramonium, Alcohol, Digitalis, Coffee |
| Netzach | Venus | Damiana |
| Hod | Mercury | Anhalonium Lewinii |
| Yesod | Moon | Orchid Root |
| Malkuth | Earth | Corn[21] |

This is just as reasonable a categorisation as any other. Especially when we consider that any categorisation is attempting to link the *chemical structure* of the drug with the *experienced effect*. Two differing interpretations of the drug material which, whilst not necessarily mutually exclusive, involve very different types of experience.

Different categorisations of drugs are useful for different purposes. One might, for example, consider drugs that cause mydriasis (pupil dilation) to be all of one type, or drugs that depress sexual arousal or whatever. Although I will be using certain broad definitions (such as 'stimulant' and 'psychedelic') below it must be remembered that these terms apply better to descriptions of the drug experience than they do to specific chemicals.

The best way to categorise drugs may well be the personal and experiential. I am familiar with contemporary occultists (and others who have explored drug effects) who have built up their own maps of drug relationships, detailing how each drug works from a personal perspective. Equally, in shamanic tribal cultures specific drugs may be related to particular animal ancestor spirits.[22]

Certainly the drugs that present most problems for classifiers are those that are vaguely grouped together as psychoactive. A plethora of terms have been used to sum up the complex effects of these chemicals - hallucinogenic, entheogenic, psychotomimetic, psychedelic etc. Lewin proposed the term *phantastica* although he admitted that it 'does not cover all that I should wish to convey.' He does not use the German term *Genußmittel*, which means 'medium or agent of enjoyment', normally applied to 'narcotics' and also 'stimulants', but which might also be applied to some aspects of psychedelic intoxication.

The type of inexpressible feeling and reactions that psychedelic drugs can provoke may lead to a transformative or numinous experience. The world is perceived as being the same yet different in our altered state. This shift in relationship with the world may be accompanied by a range of other experiences. These could include heightened sensitivity and alertness or quiet and lassitude. They may include 'distortions' of the senses and hallucinations. These changes may be felt to lie more or less inside the drug takers mind, or appear quite objective.

Again I would insist that, although most of the drugs I mention in this book are commonly known as psychedelics, any chemical, in the right circumstances can have a psychedelic action.

## Poison Years

It is worth remembering that some drugs do have quite toxic effects on the body.[23] Whilst most chemicals in sufficient amounts can permanently disrupt or stop the normal functioning of bodily systems, most of the drugs we are talking about can provide very profound effects in very small amounts. Toxic conditions or extreme stress of the chemical systems of the body (such as those produced by fasting or fever) can create experiences that are very similar to drug induced states, including the states reached by ingesting psychedelic chemicals. At the numinous peak of an acid trip,[24] one might have experiences that are paralleled remarkably with near-death experiences.

The important factor in drug experiences is that these states can be reached without going anywhere near toxic overload. Thus one of the beauties of using drugs for self transformation, for magic, is that you can stress your mind to its limit but without stressing your physical organism to exhaustion. In this sense perhaps drugs are the 'easy way out' (as they are often dismissed by the ascetic mystic) but as we've already seen, even your lofty retreat of passive meditation could be thought of as a drug. So where is the real difference in value?

Although toxic doses of certain drugs are astonishingly high (it is often, jokingly said that the fatal dose of cannabis is 2 kilos, dropped on the head from a fifth story window) much lower doses can cause massive changes in the mind that may well lead to death. In an individual with a heart condition it is not at all impossible that a strong hallucinogen could engender a heart attack, during a bad trip. Equally drugs can certainly be used, with a combination of ritual techniques (such as imprisonment, psychological and physical torture) to permanently unhinge the mind. The worst examples of these practices are inevitably from military and medical sources. These two modern industries that are so closely connected at their ideological levels (especially in totalitarian states, such as Nazi Germany) as to be almost inextricable. There are many accounts of huge doses of LSD (and many other drugs) being given in various experimental, military and medical circumstances that have certainly caused much human suffering.

In medical and pharmacological works the mental effects of any drug (especially of 'hallucinogenic' drugs) is often referred to as 'psychotomimetic'. This term suggests that this type of intoxication resembles madness. Aside of the shaky philosophical ground for this classification (after all, what is mad?) the effects of these drugs, whilst similar to 'psychotic' states do not replicate them however imperfectly.[25] There are distinct differences between the intoxication that LSD produces and that found in people with serious schizophrenia. Although there are certainly interesting parallels to be learnt between mental illness and drug states equating the two is over simplistic and serves only to brush the meaning of drug experience under the scientific carpet.

Of course madness does have its fans. For the last hundred years, and increasingly since the pseudo post-modern deification of madness, many philosophers have argued that permanent insanity is ultimate liberation (as exemplified by the insanity of people such as Nietzsche or Artaud).[26] Certainly experimentation with drugs for transformative process must require a certain sort of character, but madness is not the aim of the experiment. An individual, to participate fully in the drug experience must, in simple terms, be unlikely to flip out and permanently loose the plot. Humans are social beings. Even a personal drive towards permanent insanity can be easily described as emerging out of the culture that lunacy supposedly seeks to undermine and escape from. My feeling is that any transformative process must include what I refer to as 'the shamanic return'. That is, after gaining some new insight, some new view of the world through the transgressive experience, it must be possible to return to society and utilise that experience within a social context – to have *learned* something. What use is it if the mad utter profound truths if we, the supposedly sane, cannot understand them? If madness does have a message it must be understood and conceptualised in such a way that it can feed back into culture. This is one of the most important points concerning the special usefulness of drugs as transformative agents. The key element, but by no means the whole of the transformative story is the drug material itself. I can show you the material key to my own transformation, I can explain about the general action of the drug, I can relate my personal experiences, I can listen to you and allow for your interpretations. However if the acid I take is of such dosage, or taken in frightening conditions and I 'loose it' permanently it is unlikely that I would even understand your words, let alone desire to move toward sharing your experience. After the transgression we must be able to deconstruct the experience, to subject it to rational analysis. We must be able to see the consequences of the drug experience, to relate what it has taught us to the 'normal' reality of every-day life. Science-fiction author Robet Silverberg gives an excellent summation of the link between transformative drug experience and analysis (in the context of literature);

> A drug is a kind of magic wand; but it is a chemist's magic wand, a laboratory product, carrying with it the cachet of science. By offering his characters a vial of green pills or a flask of mysterious

blue fluid, the author is able to work wonders as easily as a sorcerer; and by rigorously examining the *consequences* of his act of magic, he performs the exploration of speculative ideas which is the essence of science fiction.[27]

## The Emperor's New Clothes

The concept of drugs straddles not only the divisions between Self and Other and between matter and mind, but also the division between natural and artificial. In fact, as we will see, the fact that drugs occupy this liminal state is part of their particular potency for transformative purposes.

In the west,[28] we tend to see the beautiful as 'natural'. Certainly since the Enlightenment a perception of nature (albeit often the carefully modelled nature of the Capability Brown landscape) as essentially good has formed. Today, for many people, artificiality has become synonymous with contrivance, affectation and of appearance but not substance. The difference in meaning and value ascribed to natural and artificial is another widely mutable concept.

For instance; vitamin C is held up as a natural material, something that will help one ward off 'flu (rather than using a 'drug' to do so). If we consume it in our diet we are taking a food supplement - a natural product not an artificial drug with a range of effects. However most vitamin C is produced in pharmaceutical factories, buildings which we would probably consider 'artificial' or possibly 'unnatural'. To eat an orange means to absorb vitamin C, this is the vitamin in its 'natural' state. Yet the same problem arises. The orange will probably be a specially selected and bred variety, it may even be genetically engineered. It is quite likely that this orange was farmed, a 'natural process' (?) and so on. Even my reason for eating it, to get my recommended intake of 'vitamin

C', relies on the existence of the human made categories of 'vitamins'. The point I am making is not that the categories 'natural' and 'artificial' are useless but rather that they are not absolute and that things like drugs play across these divisions.

Once again writers on the transformative power of drugs tend to have widely varying views on the position and relative merits of synthetic over natural substances. Leary, working in the industrialised 1960s, had no ethical problems using psychedelics that were produced in the quintessentially artificial conditions of Sandoz laboratories in Switzerland or by Oswley in illegal laboratories. It is perhaps not surprising that, for the baby boomer generation, the idea of mass-produced religious experience did not seem paradoxical.

Leary insists that: 'If you are serious about your religion, if you really wish to commit yourself to the spiritual quest, you must learn to use psychochemicals. Drugs are the religion of the twenty first century. Pursuing the religious life today without using psychedelic drugs is like studying astronomy with the naked eye because that's how they did it in the first century AD, and besides, telescopes are unnatural.'[29]

Today many neo-pagan writers, and others, want wholesome natural substances. Drugs such as psilocybin and cannabis are 'better' than laboratory made substances. This view is certainly understandable given the current importance of the political ecological movements in the west. Personally I firmly support much contemporary green politics, however there is a real danger in simplistically asserting 'nature good, culture bad'. The problem is basically that it is we humans who decide on what is, and what is not, 'natural'. To claim that there is an absolute, definable nature is to miss the point. Nature is a concept, one that plays in and out of different cultural meanings. In the 19th century most people viewed homosexuality as not only abominable in the sight of God but also as 'unnatural'. Today most intelligent people see homosexuality as no big deal. But either way it is us humans who do the defining.

In the case of drugs I agree that growing a plant that one can have a complex relationship with, that you then smoke and get high on, is a very rewarding experience. If nothing else because it exists on so many levels (one waters the plants, talks to them, strips off shade leaves and smiles as they come into bud). But I would also rather have a predictable dose of a known strength drug should I need surgery. The dosage of drugs in some plants can vary widely. In the past some occultists, such as Dion Fortune, saw this natural variation of concentrations as being one reason not to use drugs for self-transformation. So Fortune's argument, unlike that of modern Pagans, says we should avoid using hallucinogenic plants precisely because of their 'natural' variations in potency.[30]

Without a doubt there are many artificially manufactured chemicals that are today ambient in the world that are contributing to ozone depletion, asthma epidemics and cancers. However there are natural materials that do the same. The problem with human technology is that industrial societies can produce huge volumes of materials and often have a very short sighted idea of their use. When we create a new chemical, as well as asking what can we do with this stuff, we should also ask, is it appropriate to use it? What will it do to us and other species? When and how will it break down into other simpler materials and what effects will this have?

Drugs come from pre-given materials (hydrogen, carbon, nitrogen etc.) in forms that are synthesised by some plants and some animals. Indeed part of the neurochemical reason for the power of many hallucinogenic drugs relates to their similarity to neurotransmitter chemicals that occur in the brain. Yet we can create completely artificial groups of chemicals, such as the phenylalkylamines (of which MDMA is an example). These molecules do not appear to occur in 'nature' in anything like sufficient quantities to be used as drugs and would be unlikely to be discovered by anything other than modern chemistry (unlike relatively simple chemicals such as alcohol). One argument might be that we should only artificially create chemicals that already occur 'naturally'. This would mean that brewing beer would be all right but distilling alcohol would not. The problem with this attitude is that a) the distinction itself is a human construct (and therefore itself artificial), b) distillation is a 'natural' process in that it is possible according to existing (presumably pre-given) physical laws and c) who is to say that is not 'in the nature of' humans that they manufacture, along with writing, levers and gender concepts - gin?[31]

McKenna seems to suggest that the addictive features of drugs such as heroin and crack cocaine is in some sense linked to their synthetic-ness. This may be true in as much as these drugs have been subject to marketing (as consumer products) as much by governments as by criminal cartels, often covertly. Certainly there is a strong link between addictive use of some drugs and economics but this is because prohibition of any substance tends to be the political whipping boy that conveniently covers up underlying social problems. Desperate people in desperate or depressing conditions are sold heroin, television and tobacco as 'ways out' but these very things are their slavery. Not that the drugs themselves are evil, but that the problems and economic conditions created by their habitual use keep people both economically and socially disenfranchised.

Hallucinogenic drugs (such as LSD and magic mushrooms) are not usually addictive. However they can be just as much a part of an oppressed lifestyle as cocaine or heroin. The weekend raver,[32] for whom

MDMA is their only release after a week of valueless office work can be living a zombie-like existence (though this is not to deny the importance of drugs as means of recreation). The difference tends to be merely one of income. We cannot look at the poor who are addicted to heroin and conclude that heroin is itself a bad drug. Certainly the economic conditions of the world's poor, even in so-called developed nations, are truly terrible, but these are a product of oppressive societies. Our society often uses 'the drug problem' to obscure the problems of homelessness and hopelessness.

Drugs may certainly be used to oppress groups but that does not preclude them from use in the liberation of those people.

# Shamania:
# the secret history of drugs

## All Time High

Having discussed some aspects of drug experience let us look at the historical and cultural position of drugs.

Although undoubtedly open to interpretation there is convincing evidence that prehistoric cultures used drugs. Representations of psychedelic San Pedro cactus can be found on ceramics of the Nazca culture (c1000BC-AD500). Cannabis seeds have been identified in Iron age sites in the British Isles. There are images of the opium poppy in Sumerian art and in Algeria, on the Tassili-n-Ajjer plateau, rock paintings show figures sprouting what may be hallucinogenic mushrooms. Although it is difficult to tell if, in the case of Iron age cannabis cultivation, whether the plant was grown for its fibre or its 'medicinal' uses, it is likely that these were known of.

Modern ethnography of tribal cultures seems to support the view that drug use is common to all humans. Cultures without medicine, and in tribal cultures this often includes 'medicine' from transformative drug use (such as the use of morning glory seeds by the South American Zapotec people as part of divination and healing process, where the drug is not given to the patient but rather to the healer) are few and far between.

Variously termed tribal, shamanic or archaic cultures, such as those that linger into the modern period (despite the best efforts of evangelists and big business) often utilise psychedelic drugs in a social context. Not surprisingly there are many different uses of drugs in a tribal cultural setting. Sometimes the drug may be taken at an 'orgiastic' ritual, in which all members of the social group participate. In other societies only men take the sacred drug, in still others a particularly adept individual may be the sole consumer of the magic brew.[33] It is this individual that has been generalised out of many specific societies into something that ethnographers call 'the shaman'. Latterly this figure has become the convenient peg upon which all manner of quasi-new age nonsense has been hung. The word shaman itself comes from the Siberian word which, although it has come to mean a socially defined individual, might also usefully be considered as a state. To be shaman is much the same as to be a bodhisattva in that the word refers to a state of being (or 'doing') firstly and to a specific person second. Whilst I will generally refer to the shaman as a specific individual, shamanism can be best appreciated as a function of a society considered as a whole. In short, *a shamanic society is one in which its members are permitted and supported in being shaman – in transgressing and exploring the boundaries between Self and Other, between the worlds of culture and wilderness.*

One of the earliest commentators on shamanism, Mircea Eliade, says that:

> The shamanic complex is very old...The essential and definitive element of shamanism is ecstasy...the goal of the shaman is to

abandon his (sic) body and rise to heaven or descend into hell - not to let himself be 'possessed' by his assisting spirits.

By using techniques, 'technologies', that are of the body, the shaman seeks to change the world. These techniques typically include dancing, drumming, ritual drama, sex and drugs. Although some writers maintain that drug use represents a decadent phase in shamanism,[34] this view says more about our culture's anti-drugs obsession than it does any realistic cultural interpretation.

The shaman may be part of the culture as the single 'medicine man'. In other cases shamanism may be a function of the whole society, culturally accepted and validated at different times and under differing circumstances. Although we may speak of 'the shaman' we are really referring to an act. This act is essentially the transgressing or dissolving of the boundaries between human body and animal body, between heaven and hell, between subject and object, between the symbolic and the real.

The shaman (as an individual) is the 'technician of the sacred'. He or she may be a particular individual selected by accident of birth, ominous portents, early disposition or exhaustive training. Although there are examples of social castes and groups that maintain a shamanic status within a group they often do so only when they honour exceptional obligations. For instance the *mamas*, who are the ruling elite, of the South American Kogi people, must spend the first nine years of their lives in a cave before they are admitted to wider society and to the use of coca. Kept underground, with just sufficient light that they do not go blind, the mama child is fed and cared for. They are told stories of what the mother goddess has created in the world outside the cave and then, with due ceremony, are led into the light. Such a cultural practice would ensure an almost life long trip. Sustained by continuous use of cocaine, the mamas become something approaching a priesthood in the Kogi culture.

Other examples of shamanism are more diverse. Individuals from any gender and any social group may decide (in the Sioux culture) to go out on a vision quest to discover their own 'medicine'.

In western culture we tend to speak of the witch or magician rather than the shaman (perhaps because as post-modernists would point out, much of what defines the shaman is western reading of cultures of 'the other', native societies where spirituality is often seen as having a greater worth or purity than in our own society). But, in that the shaman is a person who bestrides the realms of seen and unseen, who traffics with non-human intelligences, who wealds supernatural powers and who must undergo a process of crisis and initiation – in this sense the shaman and the magician have similar goals. Some historians might argue for a distinction between the shaman and the magician. The former seeks to enter the immanent, subjective world of inner experience. The magician, through Qabalistic symbols and complex litanies, seeks to become all knowing, to have dominion over the transcendental objective world. However, I believe that these distinctions are superficial. The magician who seeks to know the mind of god must give up their own ego and even their own learning.[35] Equally the shaman must know the powers of her spirit allies and the often complex cosmology that she must navigate once beyond the mundane world.

To see shamanism as an anti-intellectual tradition and western magic as a quasi-transcendental one is to ignore that fact that both systems use very similar methods to collapse the subject/object division (or as Hofmann calls it the 'I/Thou' barrier), for very similar ends. It is like asking what defines the shape of a glove - its inside or its outside.

## Back to the Old House

During the historical period in Europe the practice of using 'visionary' drugs does seem to become less significant. Certainly when compared to South American societies, though at present there is little research as to why this has been the case.

Some writers suggest that the development of farming seems to occur in cultures at the same time as a general downturn in the use of drugs. Certainly many of the tribal cultures (especially in the Americas) who do use drugs for a whole variety of reasons (curative, initiatory, visionary, religious) often supplement horticulture with an extensive use of hunting and gathering techniques. However there are many agricultural communities who continue to make use of a large pharmacopoeia, including drugs that are used for mystical or magical purposes. Many settled communities use drug experience to support their cultural being in exactly the same way as nomadic cultures. Although settled communities may seem to exhibit less shamanic-style drug use this does not mean people in settled cultures do not need, or should avoid, drug experiences. In native farming communities there are still many examples of transgressive, visionary drug use, whilst some nomadic cultures do not use these techniques. For instance, the psychedelic Iboga is farmed by the settled peoples of the Congo and Gabon, whereas the semi-nomadic aboriginal native cultures of Australia have little or no recorded use of drugs for what in the Americas is recognised as shamanic or transformative purposes. This is despite the fact that psychoactive drugs do exist in Australia and that these cultures do have extensive pharmacopoeia for other uses.

In the Far East there are huge pharmacological traditions but little evidence of drugs being used for transformative processes (though both datura and cannabis may have featured in oriental shamanic traditions).

Instead the most common practice is the careful use of foods (remember, there is no strict boundary between a food and a drug) to balance and revitalise bodily energies. Such systems lead to modern reinterpretations of these traditions in dietary systems such as macrobiotics. In this system a very 'yang' person would be recommend to eat 'yin' foods to restore the balance of their *chi* (the vital energy of the universe as expressed through the physical body). This tradition of thinking of foods in terms of their quantity and quality of active or passive force was continued into the magical use of animal products (such as the aphrodisiac rhino horn). There is some little tradition of using magical mushrooms by Taoist monks. The chief Taoist concern in practice (though not necessarily in theory) seems to be longevity or immortality. Perhaps in these traditions the 'eternal life' spoken of by Taoist sages is as much a result of transgression through chemical gnosis (the mushrooms depicted in most texts certainly resemble some hallucinogenic species) as it is a physical longevity.

From the cultural centre the shamanic mode of human experience is pushed away to the periphery, finally to become, in Europe, closely associated with the Christian Devil and with witchcraft.

In Europe the classic picture of the village wise woman (as developed by historians such as Margaret Murray, who postulated that the medieval witch craze was centred on the lingering vestiges of a pre-Christian pagan tradition) has been vastly overstated. Yet a kernel of truth remains. The village wisewoman and cunning man can be demonstrated to have existed in some communities (in the case of famous examples, such as Essex wiseman Cunning Murrell, their existence is well documented). Equally the wandering barber surgeon and quack, share similar social positions to the tribal shaman; wandering healers, at the edges of settled communities. Whether in fact or merely in terms of iconography it is the witch who takes up the mantle of the shaman. In terms of drug use this isn't simply a similarity in the mind of the beholder since both the shaman and the witch use plants to enter trance and commune with the Other.

## Waking the Witch

During the turbulent times of Medieval Europe (the weather got colder, plague was rampant, most of the European heads of state had an average age of 19, and religious wars were frequent) the shamanic figure of the wise woman/man began to be expelled from culture. From the edge of town the witch was dragged to its centre and there examined, perhaps incarcerated and often executed. By the beginning of the modern period (when most of what we think of as the 'Medieval' witch hunts actually occurred) the witch had become the subject of the emerging judicial and parliamentary systems.

The history of the 'witch craze' is complex and surrounded by much popular lore. Figures sometimes quoted, such as 3 million women being executed during the witch trials, are beyond belief. However, it would be just as unwise to dismiss the many executions that did happen as being an series of events that did not have deep roots. History is the process of making sense out of the past and we cannot assume that the rationale of the witch-hunts cannot be interpreted. The expression 'witch craze' may suggest that we cannot understand the logic of those people who would subject others to hideous tortures for allegedly bewitching a cow. The term 'craze' seeks to distance ourselves from the meaning of the event. We do not talk of the conflicts of Catholics and Protestants as 'crazes' because they make sense, though many more people were tried as heretics and members of unpopular religions than as witches.

The fact remains, despite those books that overstate the historical evidence, that this was the persecution of witches. Those 'medicine people' who, in the archaic period were nominally within the social boundary, were ejected from culture. During the early modern period in Europe this phenomena was fixated on a number of individuals and certainly for different reasons (I am not by any means suggesting that the witches who were hunted were necessarily the village wise people). It is the allegation and belief in witchcraft, and what this meant to those involved, that is important. As in the reign of the American Senator McCarthy, it is the figure of the Communist that is ejected. You could try to pin the crime onto anyone you didn't like but it was the power and meaning of the allegation that mattered above all. It is 'the Communist' who is expelled from culture. To understand the witch 'craze' we must determine what it was that medieval culture was seeking to expel.

Witches could fly, they were fucked up the arse by the Devil, they used herbs to transform themselves, they knew secret charms and lore, they had riotous feasts with music and inverted dancing. It was this complex of ideas, a set of acts that are parallel with the transgressive work of the shaman, that were expelled from culture.

We must remember when we look at the witchhunts in Europe that we are looking at a phenomena which often had tremendous popular support (not simply a holocaust on the random poor perpetuated by the religious or economic elite). We should also note that people that we would generally recognise as 'witches' were sought out to find and deal with others of their kind. In medieval and early modern Europe, as in most other cultures, if you wanted to track down a witch the best person to hire was another witch. However this pattern does not deny the fact that, as a whole, the practices of witchcraft were in the process of being excluded from the body of society. Most notably, for our purposes, the shamanic or transgressive use of herbs (drugs).

Later, as the Enlightenment dawned, this exclusion was carried further, the birth of rational natural science sought to expunge the last traces of the shamanic or magical worldview.[36] Even when the method of science was rigorously imposed on the psychical realm that realm was denied. When in 1762 Henry Durbin,[37] a chemist and early Methodist, attempted to investigate a case of witchcraft using the scientific method his research was ignored. One could not examine such things as the demonic possession of children using the scientific method because demons did not exist *a priori*.

Many historians have suggested that from the 18th century onward, society felt that it had put the last nail into the coffin of the shamanic complex.[38] Not only had the witch trials been a mistake they had been an insanity, a 'craze'. Now society could put all that nonsense behind it and get on with the serious business of inventing such sane and reasonable systems as industrialised capitalism, colonialism and plutocracy.

The irony of this, as post-structuralists are quick to point out, is that the edifice of rational science inevitably casts the shadow of the irrational, occult and uncanny. By creating the boundaries of 'natural laws' and rational, deductive method so science excludes the 'irrational' – not until one has a concept of an orderly, mechanistic nature that can be investigated does the category of the supernatural come into being.[39]

Many groups of people today want to own the word 'witch' - feminists, neo-pagans, environmentalists[40] and others. The power of the witch today lives on as strongly as ever, we all know what witches look like -

be they the plastic hag masks of Halloween[41] or the beautiful, naked witch queens of 1970s coffee-table occult books.

Ethnographer Hans Peter Duerr, in his excellent study of social boundaries and their transgression, draws repeated attention to the fact that the witch is a creature of the borders. She is the lurker on the threshold of society, the dweller in the liminal realm. She occupies the 'null space' of Proshansky - the architect who demonstrated how, at least in English urban culture, there are a series of attitudes to space that are vitally important for planners to understand. The lift in the block of flats is a null space. It is neither defensible (personal and private, i.e. one's own flat), nor is it public (the street). It sits between the two spaces and is thus the a place for which nobody really cares for or has any attachment to. Many people have a marked hatred for these in-betweenness[42] spaces. These spaces may be imagined as physical locations but also as the psychic space between ideas or categories.

In many settled communities the shaman (or somebody who embodies more or less the aspects of this role as it appears in tribal society) lives on the edge of the world. This may be literally, in that they would dwell on the edge of a village (as does the witch in Grimms' tales, on the edge of the wild, untamed woodland),[43] or it may be a more metaphorically social 'edge'. Moreover, although farming communities may have orgiastic rituals (such as the *Lupercalia* of ancient Greece), these rituals often take place in the liminal space: on the borders of the town, or in some other sense outside the jurisdiction of 'normal' life.[44] The figure of the witch occupies this realm and, in a society such as ours that generally fears transgression, is liable to be attacked. Either the borders should be raised (by excluding the witch and making her invisible, in much the same way as lesbians have been made invisible within culture), or the offending heresy must be purged and sent packing into the wilderness.

The witch, as well as being the radical, the hedge sitter,[45] the dispossessed in-betweener, can also serve the community directly. In this case there is another strong link between the figure of the witch and that of wise-woman healer. However in order to consult her services it is necessary (usually) to visit her place, be it gingerbread cottage or hut on a chicken's foot.[46] In order to seek the assistance of the sacred realm between the worlds it is necessary, in a sense, to partake of this world oneself.

Before the 'enlightenment' it was perfectly natural to imagine that witches had power. After this time belief in witches diminishes. Samuel Johnson says that witchcraft (though perhaps real) has simply 'declined', as do many other commentators (although some forms of Christianity continue to believe in witches right up until the present, since they were part of the divinely ordained and real invisible worlds).[47] However the practice of going to the witch to seek advice was finally destroyed not by the witch trials but by the enlightenment itself. Johnson's argument that witchcraft had ceased to be a problem does not really work. What we are seeing is not the disappearance of witches but rather the disappearance of a *belief* in witches.

The trials began to fall into abeyance as the rise of secular ideologies (triumphing with John Stewart Mill's Utilitarianism) began to make the issue of personal religion less important to the state. As the historian Larner explains the witch hunts '...could not become rampant until personal religion had become political. It could not survive the advent of secular ideologies.' Indeed the witch trials themselves might be the work of the devil.[48] The act of bringing the witch into the centre of the town was like opening up a wound to the ravages of external disease. Better yet to raise the barriers, to build a cultural wall high enough that the outside of culture remained firmly excluded. There would be no more waking the witch to ask for her advice and power, we should let her sleep in story books as a fabulous and patently unreal monster, suitable only for terrifying children.[49]

## Up the Hill Backwards

The liminal symbolism of the witch (and shaman) is often expressed by their 'contrary' nature. In many cultures there are such contrary people, often with special cultural significance and powers all their own. One clear example of this is the cross-dressing 'she-males', the berdache of the Crow Indians. The berdache are men who are not men, a 'third sex'. They have special 'medicine' and serve culturally to both determine and subvert the categories of male and female. Similar she-males occur in folk tradition and esoteric symbolism, for example with the bisexual or epicene deities of Hermes, Set or Loki.[50]

The backward, contrary symbolism of the witch serves to reaffirm that she is neither subject nor object but the symbol and role adopted by those who would enter the liminal realm. Duerr points this out, saying:

> To make clear that the witch was not a being of the 'inside', that she had at least one foot 'outside', beyond culture, a reversal of the ordinary has been used since ancient times. Thus, in the *Vatnsdaela Sagai* we are told about the old witch Ljot; 'She had pulled her clothes over her head, stepping backward with her head stuck between her legs, and the glance from her eyes was not good to see, as she was casting lightning against her as a troll would.

> The witches of the Akan walk with their feet up and their heads down. The warlock (*umthakathi*) of the Zulus rides backwards on a baboon just like the witches of the late Middle Ages. Also the Yakut shaman Küstech sits astride a mountain goat, 'the hooves of which face backwards'. When the medicine man of the Western Australian Jigalong turns into his dream spirit, his *badundjari*, resembling an eaglehawk, his legs become wings, his testicles

eyes, and his anus, his beak. He flies away, his back towards the front.[51]

Because the witch is not separate from culture (she might be said to represent the *play* between notions of nature and culture) anyone might be a witch.

> In small, non-Western societies today a more 'archaic' attitude is often still encountered towards that part of the self that is sited on the other side of the fence of civilization, in the wilderness. For the Bakweri of Mount Cameroon, the world of the 'outside' is the world of the mermaids (*liengu*). This world includes the sea and the primeval forest. The 'outside' is also the realm in which the women of the Bakweri are at home…All women are outside, but the mermaids are 'more outside' than all the others. If an ordinary woman is possessed by such a spirit being…then she needs to leave the world of culture. She dresses herself in skirt made of the bark or the roots of the *iroko* tree, is given a *liengu* name and learns the language of the mermaids. After some months, at dusk, she is finally thrown into a deep waterhole by a medicine man or a medicine woman…The woman has now turned into a mermaid.[52]

The symbolism of reversal, the type of 'perverse' activity alleged of the medieval witches sabbat, resurfaces again and again in culture. In the west there is a simplistic moral overtone to the whole business. The dark, the outside of culture is defined as evil rather than as primal, as bad rather than *Bacchanalian*. Transgressive cultures in the west are instinctively drawn to the antithesis of what 'nice' society stands for. This might be the rebellious satanism of heavy metal listening youth (which, for all it is lampooned by adult society, can be a vital and empowering part of the adolescent process). The 'backwards', transgressive symbolism also appears in adult culture. For instance Albert Goldman, writing about one of the first gay dance clubs in 1970s New York, described the decor of 'salvation' as that of the Witches Sabbath. A vast painted Satan, genitals exposed and rampant, flanked by debauched angels. Drinks were served from chalices, pews set against the walls with the DJ as priest.[53] This is a perfect example of what, in occult parlance is referred to as 'tapping into the current'. In this instance the US gay scene was tapping into the cultural iconography of witchcraft. An iconography that speaks of the debauched, the hedonistic, of rude sexuality and whispers of dark perversity. Adopting the style of the transgressive need not simply be thought of as an act of rebellion, to be thought of as existing only in terms of one culture trying to turn its back on another. Tapping into the transgressive current means to forge a direct alliance with the liminal sphere. Rather than creating a culture with new (though different) norms and values, identification with the witch, with 'the dark', means to deliberately seek to shake things up.[54] As the name of the club, 'Salvation', implies liberation might well come from Satan as well as from Christ, or to use the language of the *Kulanarva Tantra* 'By what men fall, by that they rise.'

## History Repeating

Having met the shaman and the witch (our exemplars of the traveller in liminal space) let us now return directly to the subject of drug experience and throw some more commonplace assumptions about what drugs do into question.

As well as, potentially, having markedly different effects on different people (or the same person in different situations), drugs also have different effects in terms of culture. This needs to be borne in mind when using drugs for transformative purposes. Although we have documented the use of drugs for different purposes, it is sometimes difficult to reconcile these accounts with our own personal or general cultural understanding of what a given drug 'does'. For example: in Britain there is a definite cultural association between taking alcohol and violence. This manifests itself most notably in the boardroom of companies where the presence of whisky and champagne are essential to the rituals of predatory business. Equally there is the phenomenon of the 'city centre violence' in British towns and cities where young men will descend on Friday and Saturday nights to drink and brawl. In these cases the tacit link between aggression and alcohol is central. Even so, this link is not a simple causal one. Drink does not necessarily make for violence. This can be witnessed by the fact that studies in Italy[55] have shown that there is no significant cultural link, in the minds of young men in particular, between alcohol and violence. Certainly there are the same opportunities for violent behaviour in Italian towns but these are not intimately linked with drinking.

In India the Thugee cult allegedly made use of hashish as an aid to ritual murder.[56] I find simply ordering a pizza difficult enough when I'm really stoned so it's hard to imagine the same drug being implicated in this type of violence. One might argue that the de-centring effect of dope (i.e. you can loose yourself into things more easily, be it the experience of listening to music, dancing or giggling) can allow the individuals to 'get into' the frenzy of the sacrifice. Even so, we are talking about ritual murder in a sacred context and an act that needs to be performed in such a way as to permit the escape of the attackers (religions where you end up executed after your first visit to church are unlikely to attract many followers).[57]

By the same token we find that as early as 5000BC the Chinese emperor Cheng Nung recommending that his courtiers take cannabis in order to improve their attention span and memory.[58] Advice that seems to fly straight in the face of the hazy memory reported by contemporary pot-heads. Equally some drugs seem to have cultural effects that are well attested to but hard to experimentally reproduce or pharmacologically explain. For instance cocaine is, without doubt, for many people, a strong aphrodisiac. Taken nasally (rather than applied as a local anaesthetic) many male users report stronger erections, perhaps a longer period of sexual excitement before they ejaculate or even faster recovery rates. However as Robert Sabbag points out in Snow Blind;

> ...there is nothing in the chemistry of cocaine, beyond its properties as a peripheral-nervous-system stimulant and mood elevator, to indicate that it in any way enhances human sexual response - although inhaling seventy-five dollars into your bloodstream in a matter of seconds, and that at the risk of fifteen years in jail, must do something for your libido.[59]

The sexual thrill of coke certainly doesn't just apply to male users, neither is it necessary to know in advance that coke has an alleged aphrodisiac quality, for it to have that effect.[60]

The virtues ascribed to opium during the Victorian period are phantasmagorical in range. If you read books by Conan Doyle, Collins and DeQuincey you can see a wide variety of beliefs about what this drug was supposed to be capable of. Certainly we have cultural overlap with what we expect of a given drug, but I don't think it is correct to imagine the simple equation drug X = effect Y.

As another example we can look at Theophile Gautier who writes of his experiences with hashish. According to his account is seems that hashish used to be a psychedelic drug of the order we now only associate with LSD and DMT. Gautier, on smoking it, discovers;

> frenetic, irresistible, implacable laughter followed by 'fantasies of droll dreams confusedly danced about; hybrid creations, formless mixtures of men, beast and utensils; monks with wheels for feet and cauldrons for bellies: warriors, in armours of dishes, brandishing

wooden swords in birds' claws; statesmen moved by turnspit gears; kings plunged to the waist in salt-cellar turrets...[61]

As each drug emerges into use it normally goes through various phases of claims being made for it. It's an aphrodisiac (a very common claim), it makes your mind work better, it will make you stimulated, it's relaxing. There are few qualities that have not been, at some stage in history, ascribed to every drug. Cultural expectations massively influence drug experience, as shown by the historical changes in the LSD experience.

One way of imagining the effect of any drug is in terms of Buckmaster Fullers'[62] concept of *synergy*. Essentially that various elements can come together to create a situation that is more than simply the sum of its parts. A given drug is synergistic with cultural expectations, individual set and setting, method of administration and so forth. The drug experience is a complex synergy in which the drug material itself is vital, but by no means the only, part.

## When I Dream

An important consideration, when we think of any drug experience, is the role played by volition - the elusive but essential fiction of the 'I' who is having the drug experience.

Consent is vitally important in any drug experience as it is in sexual experience. Although the motivation towards transcendent experiences wells up from a source we cannot know,[63] the conscious intention to break through the limits of conventional experience by using a drug is important in dictating the direction of the experience. It is certainly possible to have spontaneous experiences of transformation (such as St Paul's vision on the road to Damascus) or experiences that one is apparently unprepared for (such as Albert Hofmann's accidental LSD trip). But in these cases the ability to successfully make the transition from 'ordinary' to 'non-ordinary' reality remains necessary. A useful drug experience (which may not necessarily be the same as an enjoyable experience) is one that the 'I' can engage with. even if this experience leads to the dissolution of the sense of 'I'.

At the peak of a trip, when the delineation between Self and Other is obliterated, the sense of 'I' becomes lost (Eliade calls this the *participation mystique*, Alex and Ann Shulgin variously term it 'The Oceanic Experience' or simply '+4').[64] The individual is one with the whole universe (or at least can discern no difference between herself and, say, the curtains). This peak can only happen if the 'I' is prepared to let go. In this sense the individual must be able to engage with the experience to the degree that he or she is willing to let 'I' cease. It is often pointed out by drug users that the surest way to a bad trip is to hang on to 'I', to be unwilling to face the dissolution of Self. This clinging to Self is the barrier to a transformative drug experience and indeed the power of drugs to undermine the habitual sense of 'I' leads to their power in areas such as psychotherapy.

The sense of self, that engages with drugs for transformative purposes, must be able to undertake two projects:

1. Letting go - deliberately engaging with an experience that will, potentially, dissolve the very sense of 'I' that seeks out the drug experience.

2. Reintegration - allowing the dissolution of the sense of self to influence and inform the new 'I' that emerges out of the experience.

In the language of Crowley's occultism, the magician must be able to give up every last drop of the sense of Self to the Chalice of 'Our Lady Babalon'[65] – to relax and, in a sense, 'die' into the non-being of Self. The magician must then have the courage to make the shamanic return to the world. This type of symbolism is central to the myth of Odin hung on the world ash tree, or Christ crucified – in order to find yourself, to undergo initiation, one must be willing to give up oneself.

The idea that 'I' can learn something by giving up 'I' is paradoxical but fits with our everyday experience. For example, I do not know how to ride a bicycle. Yet it is possible for me ('I') to learn this. Thus the 'I' that cannot ride is replaced, by the project of learning to ride, with an 'I' that can. We change our sense of 'I' all the time. For this reason the philosophical problem of what constitutes consciousness is such a huge one. 'I' am continuously changing, continuously re-creating myself into 'I's that are different from what has gone before. This process is called *autopoiesis* – literally self-creation.

Of course the 'true fiction' of 'I' has long been a thorn in the side of reductionist science, especially in the 'mental' and social sciences. As the behaviourist psychologist Watson put it, 'There is no reason why appeal should ever be made to consciousness in any of them [i.e. psychological studies]. Or why introspective data should ever be sought during the experimentation, or published in the results.'[66]

Though it is always changing, the sense of 'I' must return, it must have continuity, a story. If I'm learning to ride a bike, after the learning process 'I' must be able to make meaningful my new skill in the context of my sense of individual being. If I can learn to ride a bike, but the price to pay is to loose my sense of identity forever, then can we really say (even if it were possible for my body to somehow continue to cycle about) that 'I' have learnt anything at all?

The volition of 'I', of a sense of a purposeful autopoietic project is important when entering the world of the drug experience. Giving someone a drug, without their knowledge or without reasonable warning of its possible effects is, in my opinion, immoral. Of course, in practice one can never know what synergy will take place between a drug and an individual. However, spiking someone's beer with acid smacks of psychological rape and can be rightly thought of as an act of mental violence. A transformative experience in the case of someone who is spiked with acid is very, very unlikely. This is because the 'I', that strange voluntary fiction of the self isn't involved. Even though the drug experience can dissolve the sense of 'I', the 'I' must be deliberately involved (even if this is in the passive sense of deciding to 'go with' the experience) if the final collapse of subject and object is to be achieved in the peak moment.

## Dancing Barefoot

I believe that it is a fundamental human drive to discover who we are and who we can be. Freud and Jung refer to this process as individuation, whereas the psychologist Maslow calls this self-actualisation.[67] It is not that being authentic[68] is a desire over and above our humanity. It is not that the magician or the shaman is more than human, some kind of psychedelic *übermensch*. Rather it is the autopoietic drive that defines our humanity. Our need to be ourselves and to discover ourselves, to figure out (or at least engage in the process of figuring out) who we are is what makes us human.[69] Even though this drive can be manipulated and controlled, even though it can be censored and ignored, it will always exist as long as human history.

This drive is, I believe, identical with the process of *learning*. Not learning anything in particular but rather learning considered as a process in itself.

The educationalist Voygotsky (who worked as an educational psychologist in the former Soviet Union) developed the idea of the 'zone of proximal development'. This is an important idea that parallels the notion of the liminal space between subject and object. Essentially a zone of proximal development is a field of potential experience and knowledge that may be reached by an individual (a learner) with help and assistance. In a simple example, a child who is learning to read is able to learn by having another person help them sound out a word. By using an already known series of phonics, which are related to signs, the child can be helped into reading 'c-a-t'. In a more general sense we could say that there are things, just outside of your own understanding, but that these things lie within a field of your potential knowledge and experience. Thus, for the child, reading the word 'cat' can happen but it needs to be facilitated by something external (a teacher). However this teacher must know and be able to *play* (to teach using whatever trick is appropriate, be it phonics or 'look and say') within this field (the zone of proximal development) in order to facilitate the learning. It is for this reason that, although it is fair to think of the teacher as 'teaching reading' it is also fair to think about learning as something that happens within the individual and isn't directly causally related to teaching at all. Thus the teacher patently works through the sounds of the letters one by one - c-a-t. But when the child learns what the word is it will be for him or her self. In this sense teaching sets the scene for learning, facilitates learning, is synergistic to learning.

There is no absolute *raison d'être* for the human autopoietic drive. Certainly we can think of reasons why learning (in a general sense) is a 'good thing'. Learning to grasp objects, to talk, to fend for oneself are all pre-requisites for survival, but we should not reduce human experience to dull 'competencies'.[70] For instance; spoken language confers a number of uses but I believe the main one is simply to express our internal states to others. We don't need spoken language to hunt (wolves do well enough without it, and quiet signs would probably be better than audible words anyway). We don't need it to communicate directions (bees do that with dance), we don't need it to plan collective action (migrating birds don't need our sort of spoken language to know when to migrate). Language (audibly spoken or otherwise), which is so much part of human experience, grows from our idiosyncratic desire to tell others what we are, what we feel, what we experience.[71] If one believes in evolution[72] then self-creation and learning may confer 'advantage', but the desire to do it, the desire to learn considered as a whole, and the desire to be authentic, to transgress and to change is a defining and fundamental part of the human experience. Learning, in this sense, is not only something humans do, it is something that defines and brings us into being.

Though we can talk about self-actualisation as a 'human project', of course we actually don't know if other animals have the same, or similar projects. (Perhaps our project, as humans is to create culture which is continuously defined and subverted by technologies of transgression, perhaps for whales their form of authenticity is to sing exquisite songs.) Although the process of our individuation may be seen as springing from a cultural, rather than biological basis,[73] I firmly believe that this process is an essential component of our lived-in, embodied experience. If nothing else the very fact that we can use drugs (external, physical materials) as catalysts for the autopoietic project demonstrates that any distinction between 'biological factors' and cultural or individual factors in self-actualisation is debatable.

# Perfect Mystery: drugs, the mind and the human brain

## Science of the Gods

We may assume that mind emerges from the substrate of the brain, embodied within the organism we consider to be an individual. It must be said this is a very simplified view of the mind. But for the purposes of discussion this view of the body/brain/mind relationship is useful. Science works in 'ideal worlds' such as the mechanistic world in which Newtonian equations work out precisely, or the supposedly limited set of variables within the laboratory environment. As human beings we live in a continuum of experiences, our brains are affected by our minds, which in turn affects our body's which affect the world, which gives rise to our bodies structure, within which the brain exists and our mind is, perhaps, dependent on. If we use science we need to simplify, to limit our field of enquiry and to concentrate not on 'the whole' but on 'the part'. In this section I will be using a lot of scientific language, experimental results and theory. However I stress that this is just another language, another series of myths and symbols.

In what follows I will be examining the relationship of drug experience to human neurochemistry, neuroanatomy and pathology. The aim is to place into context the relationship between the drug as substance and drug as experience and to see where scientific pharmacology provides a good description of drug experience and where it fails.

## Happy Phantom

The human brain is beautiful, exquisitely involuted, like a complex spiral shell, composed of various more-or-less well defined areas and woven from 10,000 million neurones, packed together in a complex matrix with about 90,000 million glial cells. The entire neural system is a good deal bigger than the brain, since it incorporates the peripheral nerves (such as the receptors in our skin that permit us to feel heat, etc.), and the central nervous system, including the autonomic nervous system (the spinal cord). Moreover there are complex feedback loops that exist between the endocrine system (glands such as the adrenal, the ovaries and the thyroid) and the rest of the nervous system. Although I'm going to concentrate on the brain, and specifically the neurocortex (the so-called 'higher' brain structures) in a sense the whole of the body is a thinking system.

The number of potential connections between neurones in the brain is vast, the mathematical possibilities of neuronal connections are said to be greater than the likely number of atoms in the universe.

The science of neurology is exceedingly complex. There is some really excellent neurological research, often using very clever experiments that seek to tease apart one aspect of a cognitive process from another. However, especially in terms of drugs, much neurological research is conducted using experiments which, I feel, are both immoral and unreliable.[74]

The brain itself may well be the physical analogue of the mind in just the same way that the words on this page are the physical form of my ideas but are not themselves identical with either my mind or yours. Using this example I can change the symbols on the page and this will, in turn, give rise to different ideas in your mind - here goes: hot, shiver, nausea, Satan, chicken - the symbols change your ideas but they are not themselves identical with your ideas.

The same process might be said to take place in the brain. By changing the neurochemical (or other) functions of the brain, the mind can be altered. Indeed in our example even introducing random noise (the nonsense word, or a general disruption of the nervous system) can cause 'meaningful' experiences to arise in the mind.[75] Most drugs work by changing, in some way, the interaction between different parts of the nervous system. In a sense they are changes in the neurochemical *signs* that are the text of our minds. However these changes, like the changes of words on a page are subject to mental interpretations which can be immensely variable. Yes, this is a paradoxical view of the mind, and certainly a view that hints at dualism, but it is a paradox that I feel is supported by the evidence as I will attempt to show.

## Garden of Paradise

Let's begin by outlining a very basic model of the brain. The brain can readily be thought of as being composed of three layers, involuted or wound up on itself. The deepest level is what is sometimes refered to as the 'reptile brain'. This is the 'oldest' structure in the brain, that humans share anatomically with most other creatures. Structures like these are seen in lizards and, it is assumed, remained with our brain organisation as we evolved. The next layer up is the mid-brain, the so-called mammalian brain. Finally there is the cerebral cortex or the 'extended brain'. The cerebral cortex is usually thought of as the most recent (in evolutionary terms) and most 'human' part of the brain structure.

The extended brain is divided into two hemispheres, the left and right. These are connected by a large group of cells known as the corpus callosum. At a 'fine grain' level, the brain consists of a complex network of brain cells called neurons.

The individual neurones in the brain carry 'signals' in the form of complex chemical reactions that create a 'bow wave' of electrical current which 'flows' through the cell. The strength of the signal in a cell is constant. Moreover the movement of energy through the length of the axon can be quite slow, much slower than the passage of an electrical charge down a copper wire. When the signal reaches the end of the axon it triggers the release of a chemical messenger, a neurotransmitter. The neurotransmitter crosses the gap between one neurone and another (or several others) and the impulse is passed on. It is important to remember that this process, this chemical/electrical messaging system, does not really carry 'messages' at all. Neurones are not telephone wires carrying signals that will be 'decoded' by whoever answers the phone. This process itself, from a mechanistic perspective, is the process of thinking. There is no homunculus in the skull or, 'central meaner'[76] waiting to read or hear the messages. It is this network of changes, of firing of neurones that is the substrate of thinking itself.

The number of neurones in the brain, after we are born, is fixed. However the more stimulated the brain the more connections can be forged between neurones at the synapses. Poor diet or lack of stimulation (either internal or external) can effect the average number of synaptic connections that exist within the brain. Although the brain of a developing child or an infant is much more 'plastic' (in that the neurones are still

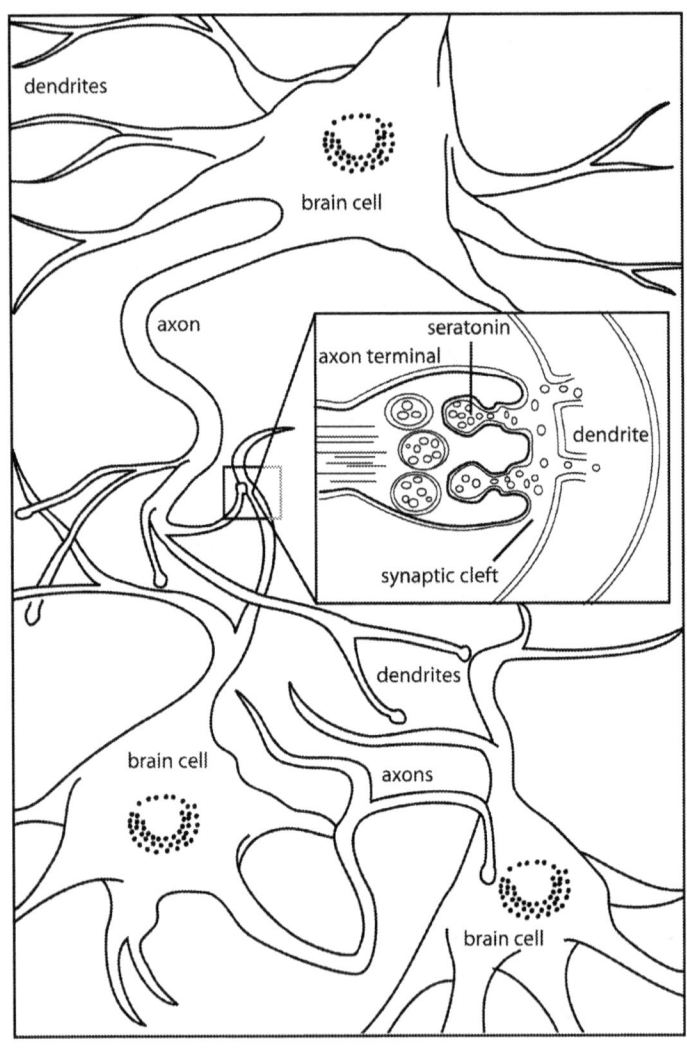

Simplified diagram of brain cells (after Saunders)

growing and dying, and connections between neurones are being formed rapidly) the system of brain synapses ensures that some degree of plasticity remains in adults.

## Last Train to Trancentral

Most drugs work by affecting the activity of the neurotransmitters at the synapses in the brain.[77] When a neurotransmitter is released from a neurone it crosses the synaptic gap and sets off a reaction in another cell. The neurotransmitter fits into the surface of the dendrite like a key into a lock. These neurotransmitters are then reabsorbed by the neuron that released them, this process is called *re-uptake*.

Drugs can change these neurochemical relationships in a number of ways. They can cause larger or smaller amounts of given neurotransmitters to be released. They may themselves mimic the molecular shape of an existing neurotransmitter, they may slow down re-uptake of a released neurotransmitter or in some other way change the 'normal' relationship between these chemical messengers.

Neurochemistry is perhaps even more fiendishly complex than neurology since it deals with a series of chemicals that are in a continuous state of flux. However for our purposes I would like to propose a huge generalisation. The neurochemical possibilities in the brain might be imagined in dualistic terms, providing us with a kind of model 'yin' and 'yang' of neurochemical relationships.

The first is the chemical that is implicated in what we usually think of as catabolic, the second with anabolic processes. In drug neurochemistry the two main chemicals that feature are serotonin (catabolic - yin) and dopamine (anabolic - yang). In fact these chemicals are more like points upon a wheel than polarised extremes. I could have chosen other dualities of systems within neurochemistry but these two transmitters are perhaps the most well researched and interesting from the point of view understanding the effects of many commonly used drugs.

Since the human body maintains itself in some kind of balance (or homeostasis) these neurotransmitters are actually part of an on-going cycle of chemical, electrical, glandular, dietary, and other interactions. Indeed one might realistically think of drug effects as being a function of homeostasis, in other words the body is not under stress when we trip anymore than when we break wind from eating too many beans. A 'trip' is the body's way of maintaining homeostasis, incorporating and metabolising material whilst producing 'side effects' – perhaps including stimulation, hallucinations or whatever.

Our simplified model of a neurochemical dualism is, of course, open to great deal of criticism but it is valid in three ways. Firstly, that neurology is very complicated and most of the data collected to date simply doesn't add up to anything like a coherent picture. So by overlaying a series of hypotheses about neurochemical relationships we may learn something about these relationships, and indeed notice the points at which our simplistic model breaks down.

Secondly, it is a way of summing up the neurochemical effects of a whole range of subtle, interactive chemical systems. A tool for explanation which relates neurochemistry to perceived drug experience at a psychological level.

Thirdly, I believe even this very simple model can help us make predictions about the effect of drugs.

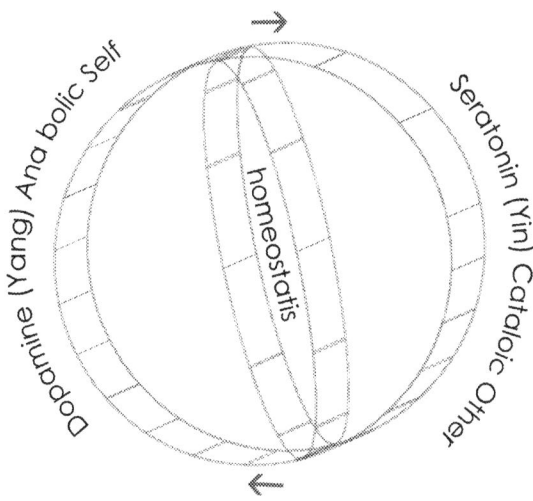

Before we examine the relationship of serotonin and dopamine, I want to set the scene by examining some of the other 'dualist' systems that are fundamental to neurology.

## Top of the World

As mentioned above, the cortex, the 'human brain' tissue, consists of two major hemispheres. This feature has lead to a whole range of experiments and investigations that is known as the study of 'cerebral lateralisation' - that is the apparent way that certain mental processes are focused more on one or other hemisphere. Much has been written of the 'specialities' of each hemisphere, including some really broad generalisations. Even so there is much to be gained by looking at the model of the brain (and its extension into the mind) which cerebral lateralisation provides.

Almost all animals show some degree of cerebral lateralisation (in fact some rather sad experiments show that 'oblation', that is the destruction of the left-hemisphere in birds, stops them singing). Although in most people one hemisphere is usually said to be 'dominant' (or 'lead'), for language either hemisphere can fulfil this role. Much of the research into cerebral lateralisation is drawn from studies of patients who have undergone commissurotomy, which is the process of severing the bundle of nerve fibres (the corpus collosum) that connects the hemispheres together.

Research by Geschwind[78] claims that the right hemisphere seems to develop first in humans and the left hemisphere slightly later. The area of the cortex on the left is generally slightly greater than the right.

Although it is important not to see cerebral lateralisation as a strict division of function, we may make certain generalisations about the activity of the different hemispheres based on scientific studies. These

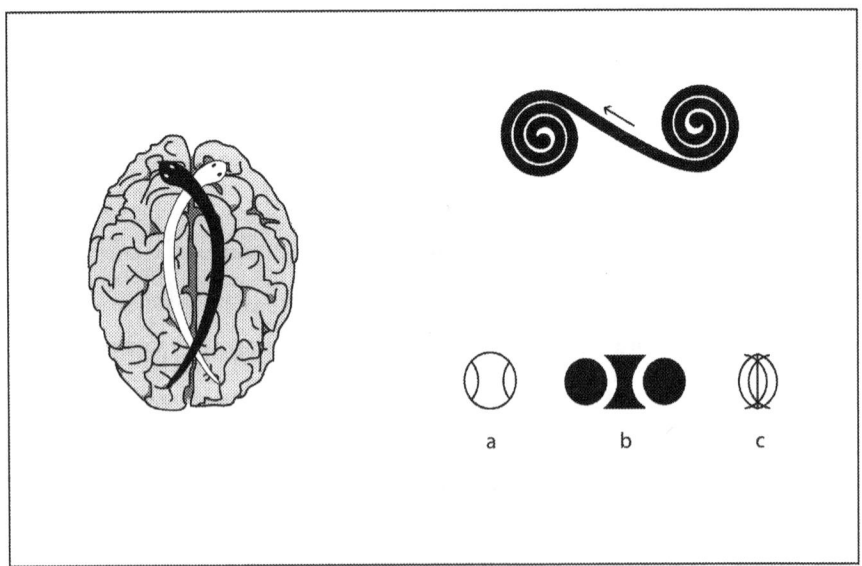

Examples of bilateral brain motifs from Desana people

studies, interestingly, parallel a number of esoteric and folk doctrines, especially where the role of cerebral lateralisation in terms of 'handedness' is concerned. They also directly parallel a number of shamanic interpretations of brain form and function, for example the Desana people studied by Gerardo Reichel-Dolmatoff.[79]

One hemisphere (in most people the left one) 'rules' such aspects as logical, sequential, verbal abilities. The other (usually right) deals with mathematical ability, spatial function, and non-verbal experiences.

Thus to generalise still further one might reasonably say that one hemisphere deals with 'parts' (sequences) and the other with 'wholes' (or 'gestalts'), it is perhaps too general to talk of a 'logical' and 'emotional' role on the part of each hemisphere, but this basic duality remains true. In essence, one part of the brain seems connected with analysis (into parts) and the other with synthesis (into wholes). A neurological version of the alchemical axiom *solve et coagula*.

For instance we might describe the relationship of the two hemispheres as a polarity or 'dichotomy'. Human culture is full of such dichotomies, and so it's perhaps not surprising that we find these appearing in neurology. Here are some instances of dual systems after the work of Robert Ornstein:

| | |
|---|---|
| Many sources | Day / Night |
| Blackburn | Intellectual / Sensuous |
| Oppenheimer | Time, History / Eternity, Timelessness |
| Deikman | Active / Receptive |
| Polanyi | Explicit / Tacit |

| | |
|---|---|
| Levy, Sperry | Analytic / Gestalt |
| Domhoff | Right (side of body) / Left (side of body) |
| Many sources | Left hemisphere / Right hemisphere (of the brain) (of the brain) |
| Bogen | Propositional / Appositional |
| Lee | Lineal / Nonlineal |
| Luria | Sequential / Simultaneous |
| Semmes | Focal / Diffuse |
| *I Ching* | The creative; heaven / The Receptive; earth |
| *I Ching* | masculine, Yang / feminine, Yin |
| *I Ching* | Light / Dark |
| *I Ching* | Time / Space |
| Many sources | Verbal / Spatial |
| Many sources | Intellectual / Intuitive |
| Vedanata | Buddhi / Manas |
| Jung | Casual / Acasual |
| Bacon | Argument / Experience |

...and so forth.

Once we have a model (i.e. specialisation of the cerebral hemispheres) any duality will fit into it. Many of the simple assertions about the role of right and left hemispheres are undermined by detailed scientific research. Yet the essential point still stands; that the different aspects of our mental process are described by science as 'happening' in different structures within the skull.

Of course this may well tell us more about the way the western mind works than anything about the objective structure of the brain. But let's continue to use the language of science and look closer at the phenomena of laterialisation, especially those aspects that can be compared to folklore about the mind.

## Halfway to Crazy

In most people the left hemisphere is dominant for language and controls the right hand which is the 'favoured' hand. A complex network of evidence demonstrates a strong link between handedness and cerebral lateralisation. Handedness is a continuous phenomena rather than a discontinuous one. In other words an individual may well be right-handed for some things, left-handed for others. Most people show a mixture of handed preferences. Interestingly writing is the most right-handed of right-handed functions. People who have a left hemisphere that is dominant for language will almost always write with their right hand. In fact the percentages from experimental work show that writing is perhaps one of the most reliable ways of gauging cerebral dominance.

There may well be some slight inherent predisposition for the left hemisphere to be dominant for handedness. Through factors that occur during gestation (such as slight hormonal changes or even foetal damage) either 'random' or right hemisphere dominance can result, but this is not by any means to say that left-handedness is always the result of 'damage'.

A more invasive way of looking for cerebral dominance (within a given task) is to use an intracarotid injection of sodium amytal. This practice, known as the Wada test, works by anaesthetising one hemisphere of the brain. Generally the patient is asked to raise both arms and start counting. Let's assume that the left carotid artery is injected, putting the left hemisphere to sleep, in this case the patients right hand will drop and she will stop counting and remain speechless. In a very high percentage of people, (about 95% of those who write right-handed and over half those who write left-handed) this suggests that certain aspects of sequential thought (in this example, counting aloud in spoken language) or at least verbal output, is in some way connected with left hemisphere activity.

Although the right hemisphere cannot speak it does not follow that it cannot think, indeed it may well be that the right hemisphere provides the foundation for thought and the left the expression of thought in a sequential manner. The neurologist Michael Gazzanigna says 'There is some final system, which I happen to think is in the left hemisphere, that pulls all this information together into a *theory*...and that theory becomes our particular theory of ourselves and of the world.'

There are individuals who do not show a distinct cerebral specialisation. Indeed studies of neuropathology show that, if the brain is damaged, say by a stroke or other injury, some functions can be transferred from one hemisphere to the other.

There is a long and diverse folk tradition that identified the left hand as being 'strange'. Indeed the word sinister means literally 'to the left' and the symbolism of left-handedness and its cultural meaning are often connected with the non-verbal world that many drugs (especially psychoactive drugs) allow us to access. This association of strangeness is the same as the contrary or backward symbolism of the liminal shaman.

Folk tradition claims that the world of the right hemisphere, of the 'left hand path', is in some way odd, perhaps to be feared or specially respected. Twins show a high degree of left-handedness, and indeed left-handedness seems to be more common in people who have some form of brain damage or anomaly (like the shaman of old, such 'damaged' people may even be called 'backward' or at least 'gauche'). This is, of course, not to say that left-handedness is inherently pathological or 'weird'.

Cerebral anomalies can include 'the pathology of genius'. For instance, a very large percentage (much higher than a random population sample) of artists and architects are left-handed. One theory is that damage or early influences on hemisphere development, that retard the usual dominance of the left-hemisphere, mean that the individual brain compensates by creating right-hemisphere dominance. This can provide the individual with special abilities; perhaps the increased visio-spacial awareness (as architects must develop) or a highly developed appreciation of pattern (as mathematicians require).

Once again the folk tradition asserts that a strangeness, and perhaps even a wounding (for instance, brain damage or the general fact that left-handers tend to have a less robust immune system), is a pre-requisite for special 'psychic' skills or genius. All this may be supported by neurological data.

## Insane in the Brain

The effect of drugs in relation to cerebral lateralisation also shows some interesting features. For instance in people who suffer from bipolar disorder (manic-depression) the salt lithium can be used to treat the condition. Although there is some uncertainty over how lithium works it may be due to an equalising effect across the two hemispheres. Bringing them together into one whole, rather than two individuals who swing wildly between sleepy depression and exaggerated excitement.

In a 'normal' person we still experience moments when the activity of the hemispheres gets out of sync. An example of this might be doing something that makes sequential sense but is, considered as a whole, inappropriate. Putting the milk in the oven and the roast dinner in the refrigerator might be thought of as an instance where the left hemisphere of the brain has achieved momentary dominance - the sequence makes sense (opening the fridge, placing the object inside, shutting the door) but the whole picture, the gestalt, is incorrect. Generally the right-hemisphere is silent, although conditions such as dyslexia, where the writer puts the letters on the page but in an inappropriate order, could be seen as being due to an 'over activity' of the right hemisphere.

One important situation in which the right hemisphere is far from inactive is during drug experience. It is common, for instance during an acid trip, to find the sequential world of TV or writing meaningless; whereas a new depth is experienced in music or complex patterns and mandalas are seen in closed eye visual hallucinations. What were previously 'random' phosphenes[80] (the colours we see when our eyes are closed) are resolved into cartwheels of colour or even alien cityscapes. Indeed the effect of LSD on commissurotomy patients is marked - they do not trip! Or perhaps it would be more accurate to say that the experience of tripping that is occurring in the right hemisphere cannot be verbalised (because the corpus collosum connecting the hemispheres is cut) through the speaking left-hemisphere. This finding is remarkable since it suggests that LSD might provide a method for 'turning up the volume' of right-hemisphere perception. Certainly LSD does make the world look 'strange' or even 'sinister'. Moreover the observation that, during the majority of the LSD trip, there is a sense that you *know* that you are tripping, may be precisely because the left-hemisphere has had to take a back-seat but remains active. In other words the gestalt perceiving right-hemisphere has, temporarily, become dominant, but the left-hemisphere, the language brain, knows that the experience is due to the drug.

It would be interesting to see if other drugs have a more or less specific action on one or other hemisphere. Certainly the very fact that we know a drug experience to be such, suggests that the feeling of the hit (be it from cocaine or THC) is registered primarily in the right-hemisphere and understood (made into a theory as Gazzaigna puts it - i.e. 'I'm having drug experience') in the left-hemisphere.

This returns to my earlier suggestion that drug experience gives us access to a different realm, the realm of sensation and of gestalt experience, but that in order to learn from a drug experience, our rational, sequential mind must be involved too.

## Body and Soul

Descartes famously placed the physical location where matter and mind interact within the pineal gland. This part of the brain is undivided (unlike the extended brain). It is easy to locate in children (being pine-cone shaped and near the roof of the third ventricle of the brain). As we age it tends to become fibrous and encrusted with calcium. In some individuals it is almost entirely atrophied.

The role of the pineal gland within the neurochemical or endocrine systems of the body is poorly understood. What we do know it that this gland responds directly to activity in the optic nerves. Indeed in some species the pineal is a properly light sensing system (as it is in some fish). Because of this responsiveness to light the gland is sometimes known as the third eye - another aspect of neurology that has direct resonance with a more esoteric view of the body.[81] One thing that the pineal gland certainly does do is to secret melatonin. Melatonin is the precursor to a number of neurotransmitter substances (among them serotonin). It is also connected with skin pigmentation and its production is influenced, at least in part, by light.

Melatonin tends to be released during the hours of darkness.[82] Certainly melatonin, taken orally, is a wonderful anti-insomniac. Melatonin production may be connected with dreaming since the effect of taking melatonin orally is to provide a good night's sleep but often one coloured by very vivid dreams. Accounts from drug users on the internet report that melatonin, taken with drugs called MAO inhibitors, can create what one writer describes as 'waking dreams'.[83] I've conducted experiments with melatonin myself and think that it might prove useful for inducing lucid dreams. These are dreams where the individual becomes conscious that she is dreaming from *within* the dream state. The use of MAO inhibitors prevents melatonin being rapidly metabolised in the body, which releases the hallucinogenic potential of this drug. A vital point here is that melatonin occurs endogenously (i.e. within the body) but through synergy with an MAO inhibitor provokes a significant drug experience.

The effects of psychedelic melatonin parallels the chemistry of the 'vine of the soul' used in South American shamanism. The preparation *ayahuasca* contains the alkaloids harmine and harmaline and the powerful hallucinogen dimethyltyptamine (DMT). Harmine and harmaline are both beta-carbolines which are themselves hallucinogenic at close to toxic concentrations.[84] However they can be used at lower levels to prevent the enzyme systems of the body breaking down DMT (which is normally inactive, as a hallucinogen, when taken orally, much like melatonin). Harmine is found in Syrian rue, which was the plant generally used by people experimenting with drugs (according to accounts on the internet) to potentise their over-the-counter melatonin pills into a powerful psychoactive. So we are left with the following strange pattern. Namely that melatonin (which is itself chemically related to DMT, which also occurs endogenously) can produce magical hallucinations. When combined with an MAO inhibitor this could potentially trigger a numinous drug experience.

The relationship of melatonin to human pigmentation again parallels folklore. Strange colouring, such as red hair or albinoism may well be connected with 'special powers' (culturally this can be anything from prodigious ability through to magical skills and second sight).

There is a link between odd eye pigmentation, left-handedness and what is called delayed 'neural crest migration' in the developing foetus. The odd colouring of the person selected to be the tribal shaman may be an observable way of determining an individual who has a higher than normal level of melatonin in their body. Such an individual might well dream more deeply, be more susceptible to lucid dreams and might well have some special ability that would be of cultural significance (like being able to speak to spirit ancestors in their dreams).[85]

Perhaps Descartes was right to suggest the pineal gland as the link between spirit and matter.[86] The experience of profound drug intoxication (such as those possible with ketamine, DMT or Thornapple) is of an 'artificial reality', just the sort of reality we experience on a nightly basis in dream sleep. The idea that dreams carry with them some form of meaning is supported by both esoteric opinion, folklore and psychoanalysis, and recently by research into memory and REM sleep by neurologists. Perhaps the pineal body might be an endogenous key to transformative states and even whole new experiential realms from which knowledge can be obtained.[87]

The mysterious activity of the pineal gland also serves to show how the brain is emphatically located in the world. Not only does this gland have a role in regulating the 'internal clock' and processes such as sleep, but it responds directly to the light and darkness. We should remember, even in the minutiae of neurochemistry, that the brain is within the body and the body within the world. The process of thinking takes place within a network of relationships, activity and meaning – not alone in the 'black box' of the brain. Even the idea that we are individuals is a dubious one in that we might better be thought of as a company (or 'conspiracy' as the occultist Pete Carroll puts it)[88] of cells. These cells include the fauna and flora of our guts and the semi-autonomous mitochondria bodies that inhabit cells.

Where we choose to draw the line between Self and Other, between matter and mind is always open to doubt, interpretation and 'play'.

## I'll be Your Mirror

So to sum up the above we can say that drugs, in most but not all cases, alter the movement of neurotransmitters between cells. We can further say that the effects of drugs can vary depending on their selective activity on different hemispheres of the brain (given our simplistic model of their functional specialities). In most right-handed people the left hemisphere is dominant for verbal skills and in some left-handed people the right hemisphere is dominant. The expression of right-hemisphere dominance, as left handedness, is often associated in folklore with special abilities or illness. Moreover we can say that the example of the pineal gland shows how the brain is intimately linked outwards to the world (through its sensitivity to light) and that the brain should not be simply considered as a 'thinking machine', in isolation, within the skull.

Finally we can say that there are remarkable parallels between folklore, occultism and the ideas of neurology. That the shaman, who 'draws on the right-hand side of the brain', should also be the 'wounded healer' and perhaps albino, starts to make more sense. The fact that a powerful psychedelic such as LSD should primarily affect the right-hemisphere might suggest that the phenotypic (that is observable characteristics - such as odd eye pigmentation) traits that are commonly displayed by the shaman are a way of guessing that such-and-such an individual may have more access that most to the 'strange' right hemisphere aspects of consciousness. It may be that the person identified as shaman will be more competent, more predisposed to moving in the melatonin/right hemisphere world of drug induced dreaming. In another sense, it could be that for all of us, right or left handed, becoming the shaman means switching off from our left-hemisphere sequential processes and focusing on the gestalt knowledge of the right side of the brain.

So we have a polarity of neurotransmitters, serotonin and dopamine, we have a dual model of hemisphere function based on cerebral lateralisation. The presence of endogenous hallucinogens in the brain, and their possible production in the pineal gland has been identified. Also we have seen that the brain is intimately related to the environment and not an isolated entity.

# Odditorium:
# the dual process of the mind

### Hell is Round the Corner

Now let us examine a duality in behaviour that serves as a model to link together neurochemical processes on the one hand, and lived-in human experience on the other. These two 'conditions' have been the subject of much attention by neurologists, doctors, psychologists and psychoanalysts. There are schizophrenia and autism. These illnesses show how, by admitting the existence of human experience to clinical and neurological data, we can find fuller ways of understanding 'mental illness' and a better understanding of the use of drugs as a therapy.

With autism nobody can hear you scream, but with schizophrenia everybody can. Neither of these conditions should be glamorised. If nothing else, if you talk to people with either condition or observe their behaviour it becomes all too obvious that much of their 'madness' is the result of a perfectly understandable sense of fear. They have difficulty relating to others, their language (if they have any spoken words) can seem flat and monotone (much like the speech of commissurotomy patients). They seem to lack emotion or to be provoked into blind rage by minor changes in their routine.

Although nobody is sure how autism occurs (the fashionable theory that it is genetic, as with so many other things)[89] the effects can be profound. In severe cases the autistic person will sit soundlessly rocking, apparently unable to interact in a normal social setting. They may develop obsessive rituals. Some may demonstrate 'special abilities'. The so-called *idiot savant* or person with Asperger's syndrome[90] might be able to memorise an entire city's bus time table, but be unable to catch a bus and go shopping. She (although it is more frequently he) cannot understand that another individual does not know what they know. For this reason the autistic person may throw a tantrum when they are told to finish their drink when they have already done so.

There are degrees in autism and many people who are very mildly autistic function quite well in the mainstream world. Indeed there are institutions in our society (most notably the high levels of crack military units) where a form of encultured autism would be valuable.

Although autism is usually diagnosed with a check list of criteria it is a definite 'complex'; a pattern of symptoms that betray the existence of a real condition. One standard diagnostic criteria includes the following symptoms.

- Qualitative impairment of reciprocal social interaction.

- Qualitative impairment in verbal and non-verbalcommunication, and in imaginative activity.

- Markedly restricted repertoire of activities and interests.

(After the international Classification of Diseases issued by the World Health Organisation).

## Imagine...

Autism in general terms could be thought of as a lack of imagination. The autistic person cannot imagine what it is like to be another person; to have thoughts, feelings, secrets that are *similar* to, but *different* from their own. People with autism, who have been able to convey the inner feeling of their condition, have repeatedly said that it feels as though everyone else has a sort of telepathic ability. Other people (according to the autistic individual) seem to 'know' what others are thinking. Imagine for a moment what it is like to have severe autism. The world appears random, strange and terrifying. Your only solace is order (be it the sequence of life, usually highly regimented to make residents of care homes happier or the order of prime numbers). Everyone else, if you can even perceive them as being like you, seems to share a secret understanding. At worst they appear as strange monsters who do nothing that makes any sense.

Autism can only be diagnosed with any certainty, over about the age of four. It is after this age, according to most child psychologists, that the child develops a personality (in the technical sense) and breaks through what I call the 'imaginative discontinuity'.

Psychologists have performed a fascinating range of experiments to investigate the imaginative discontinuity. Generally speaking children under the age of three, however good their verbal skills, are unable to understand how another persons perspective would be *similar to* but *different from* their own experience.

As an example; an autistic child is shown a tube that normally, would be expected to contain sweets. The psychologist then demonstrates that the actual content of the tube is a pencil. Now if another person comes along and the child is asked what that other person will imagine to be in the tube they will usually reply 'a pencil'. There is no concept that the contents of the mind of another person might not include information present in the mind of the autistic child.

The difficulty for autistic people is that they do not fully break through the imaginative discontinuity. They do not develop the ability to *imagine* other minds as similar and yet different, and to imagine the contents of another person's mind might contain either less than they know about a given situation, or indeed more. This is a subtle, but in practice, often tremendously debilitating state of affairs. Indeed the fact that so many people with autism function so well in the world is a testament to the fluidity and adaptability of the human mind.

## Strangers

The ability to commit a bus timetable to memory but not to catch the bus sounds like an example of left hemisphere dominance. In it we see the ability to sequence, to 'process' information in an analytical way, to structure and store it in memory. The information can also be recalled, frequently with lightning speed.[91] Even so, the whole purpose of this information (to allow the person to get on the right bus, at the right time, to go to the right place) is forgotten. Equally the telepathy which autistic people feel the rest of society possesses is just the sort of 'hallucination' that often accompanies right-brain, 'gestalt' focused stimulation (such as that produced by psychedelic drugs). It is exactly this realm of meaningful 'wholes' that the autistic person is excluded from.

Interestingly there are cases of autism being 'cured', sometimes by autistic people themselves. One case concerns an individual with Aspergers syndrome (unusually mild autism often coupled with high intelligence and often exceptional ability in one or more fields) who created a cradle to squash his body. After using this device he found his autism greatly reduced. Perhaps we might think of this as a deliberate attempt to force the mind to recognise (and thus imagine) relationship in a direct physical way. Although autistic people do not often like to be hugged they often enjoy being tightly tucked into bed or in some other way closely covered. For 'normal' people the experience of being hugged leaves us feeling wanted, comforted and happy - for people with autism it can also be part of a genuine therapy. Physical 'holding therapy' has been used, with some success, in treating autism.

If anyone finds it difficult to transgress the boundaries of the self it would seem to be people with autism. In fact there are some additional features of the condition that throw light on the whole thesis of transgression. One is that their condition (and the panic behaviours which it results in) are often quelled by quite different mixtures of drugs. For some, powerful tranquillisers will have no effect, while others will find the smallest amount of stimulant will have devastating results (such as hypertension). This difference in drug susceptibility may in part be due to difference in neurochemical mix and cerebral dominance. This does not necessarily mean that the *brain* of the autistic person is 'wired' in a radically different way to 'normal'. What it does mean is that the *mind* of people with autism is quite differently constructed compared with those people who are fortunate enough to have crossed the imaginative discontinuity. What we must always remember, when considering the action of drugs, is that they are primarily *experiences* and it is certainly true that the experience of the world is quite different for people with autism.

The autistic can become psycho-physically 'stuck',[92] unable to transgress, to learn with the ease that which post-imaginative people can. An autistic person might repeat the same word again and again, relieving anxiety through sequential repetition, and perhaps desperately searching for *meaning*. As well as seeking solace in routine or reciting number one hits from 1982 onwards, they also become stuck *within* this knowledge. They cannot transcend it into the world of meaningful data. They have a skill (e.g. knowing the bus timetable by rote) but this knowledge cannot be 'transferred', it cannot be made meaningful or useful in a broader context. They are trapped in a world of data without being able to use that data as information.

Autistic people sometimes become physically 'stuck' in doorways or other borderline spaces. This is an embodied expression of the inability to 'translate', to transgress, to move knowledge (or the physical body) from one domain (or location) to another. The autistic person becomes frozen on the liminal threshold, unable to transgress and change their bodily position. A strange behavioural symptom of a psychological lack.

## Rage against the Machine

As autism represents a lack of theory of mind (i.e. that other minds exist and are similar yet different), and a disconnection from the social world, so schizophrenia is an often terrifying encounter with the 'SuperReal'.[93] People who suffer from schizophrenia commonly suffer from hallucinations which are similar to (though quite distinct from) those encountered during psychedelic experience. These hallucinations can vary from mild distortions of the world, to whole nightmarish episodes which, unless you have taken psychedelics and experienced a 'difficult trip', are hard to imagine.

One of the most common experiences for the person with schizophrenia is audio hallucinations - hearing voices. These are often reported as being as clear as 'actual' spoken words. These voices may appear to come from objects or to be completely discarnate. They may change continuously or, more often, come from various 'entities'. These symptoms naturally cause the person with schizophrenia to look for an answer to the changes in the world around them (since schizophrenia generally begins around puberty). This often leads to a complex set of delusions about the world (the schizophrenic may believe that he or she is endowed with special powers, mystical insight or the subject of special reward or punishment from God). They are left trying, as one schizophrenic person expresses it, to make a universe in which 'Everything had to be connected up somehow...I had to make sense out of it all and connect it up with what I was trying to do with my life.' The drive, to make sense of a universe riddled with hallucinations and strange messages that only the schizophrenic person seems to hear, naturally enough, often drives people insane. Schizophrenia can easily lead to acute paranoia and thence to violence, self-harm and perhaps suicide.

Schizophrenic symptoms can also include catatonia, '...abnormal movements as distinguished from abnormal thoughts and speech...assuming a fixed, often uncomfortable posture and remaining motionless for an extremely long time.'[94] This ability to sit motionless is an often aimed for ability within belief systems that require endurance (such as Native American Shamanism) or profound concentration (such as Zen meditation or yoga). Strangely this trance-like state can include 'waxy flexibility where the body of the schizophrenic person will hold any pose that it is put into. If a carer raises the schizophrenic persons arm, whilst they are in a catatonic state, they will hold their hand up indefinitely. Catatonia can also include 'excessive, purposeless and disorganised movements,'[95] these can be violent flailing or can range through any number of 'strange' behaviours. Wearing clothes in a socially inappropriate manner, grimacing in front of mirrors, removing clothes and so on. Removing one's clothes is a behaviour that can be provoked by psychedelic experience. Intoxication with datura, the powerful psychedelic thornapple, often leads to the user removing his or her clothing.[96] In catatonia the paradox of drug experience and effects emerges, as it does in autism. An injection of a small amount of barbiturate (which normally induces relaxation and sleep) will release a motionless catatonic person from their statue-like stance.[97]

## The Subtle Energies Commission

In the Hermetic tradition of Western occultism there is an initiation called the Master (or Mistress) of the Temple. At this initiation the candidate makes a 'magical oath' to 'interpret every act of the universe as a direct dealing of God with my soul'.[98] For someone with schizophrenia they have, involuntarily and often permanently, taken just such an oath. The voices that the schizophrenic person hears are not just the background hubbub of thought, they are often direct injunctions, responses (apparently external) to un-said thoughts and feelings. Moreover, things in the world that are not particularly significant cease to have either a general sense of meaning or perhaps irrelevance. Information (words, objects, events) cannot be shut-off as just redundant background noise. One person with schizophrenia expressed this predicament by saying that;

> It was a sinister feeling of meanings locked behind meanings. A lamp was not just a lamp; it had a personality and it was trying to communicate with me. A chair was not just a chair, it seemed more real than reality itself. It scared me. I thought that I was approaching some kind of horrible Enlightenment about which I felt quite ambivalent. I walked around feeling as if I was exposing the

barrenness of my soul before God; the fact that everyone could hear all my most private thoughts did not help either.⁹⁹

The telepathy which excludes the autistic person, is unbearably present for the schizophrenic.

So as autism is to be cut off from the world, to be schizophrenic is to be exposed unendurably to it. There is no privacy, no 'also rans' in perception. Every internal thought is scrutinised by voices, everything has profound and personal meaning.

Perhaps one of the most interesting things is the way in which many schizophrenic people focus their fears on electrical equipment. Fear of the radio, the notion that the electric toothbrush is sending out deadly radiation, and the idea that TV broadcasts contain information specifically for the schizophrenic viewer.

The perception that TV broadcasts contain hidden messages, that only the schizophrenic person can see or hear, is quite common. So too is the idea that TV can be directly interactive. The reporter might pause, whilst reading the headlines, to tell the schizophrenic not to pick her nose. The idea of the invisible force (the telepathy that autistic people say seems to operate on the part of non-autistic individuals) is common in schizophrenia. Sometimes this emerges as the belief in an omniscient, far reaching conspiracy, sometimes as the machinations of god or the devil, sometimes as invisible radiation (which the schizophrenic person may believe that they must protect themselves from in order to stay sane). It is perhaps the fact that in modern culture we *do* have external, disembodied voices (in the form of radio and television) that makes electrical equipment the focus for many schizophrenic delusions. Rather than being general information fed to the world at large (such as the Ten o'clock News) the broadcast is specifically for the schizophrenic individual and may contain hidden messages and meaning.

## Bodystealers

The historian Julian Jaynes has suggested that, until quite recently, human beings did not conceptualise their voluntary thoughts as being 'internal'. By a close reading of the Iliad, Jaynes comes to the conclusion that there was no 'I' (in the sense we use it) within ancient European culture. His argument is that ancient humans, like modern-day schizophrenics, literally heard commands issuing from statues of their gods. The notion of volition did not emerge until quite recently (in the classical period), before this, it was not so much that 'I' might seek to kill Hektor but rather that 'the gods' ('the Voices') told me to.

Although it is difficult to accept the pre-Classical 'bicameral mind' (as Jaynes calls it, before the narrative centre of 'I' emerged) as representing an absolute discontinuity, there is certainly merit in his hypothesis. If nothing else, although we scarcely admit it, today much of what any 'normal' person does are things that they are 'told' to do by an agency that we externalise but that is usually thought of as internal. At one end of the scale there are the tremendous number of people who regularly experience audio hallucinations but manage to avoid being called 'mad'. Even amongst those who have had problems dealing with this experience there are those who have used their 'delusions' in a variety of creative ways. For example, the singer/songwriter Kristen Hersch[100] 'hears' the songs that she writes as fully formed pieces, with melody and lyrics. Although herself subject to the problems that the label 'mentally ill' can bring with it, she is able to channel her 'voices' in a remarkably creative and positive way. Equally, on a day to day basis, many people externalise their inner feelings. We speak of aspects of our consciousness in terms of independent entities (our 'intuition', or 'conscience', which may well be represented as a miniature figure, the angel or devil on one's shoulder). We project our own feelings onto others (as the therapist may see dramatically in psychoanalysis), we may externalise our sexuality (the phenomena is particularly obvious in men who may name their penis and ascribe to it 'a life of its own').

## Come Together

My use of autism/schizophrenia as a dual model of mental states should not be taken as an absolute duality. There are many differences that mean that these conditions should not be read as absolute opposites. Chiefly is the fact that, although some schizophrenic people relate having hallucinations before puberty, the autistic individual is (usually) born with their disability whereas for the schizophrenic it (generally) only emerges around their teens.

Another important point is that many of the same symptoms are shared by schizophrenia and autism. This is hardly surprising. since both conditions represent mental states that are radically different from the accepted norm. It is hardly surprising that people who have these conditions should attempt to protect themselves from the hostile world in similar ways. Lack of communication, withdrawal, violence, repetitive or ritualistic behaviour - these reactions are not necessarily part of the schizophrenia or autistic complex. We can see this in our own everyday experience of stress (sulking, aggression, chain smoking etc.). Many of the features previously believed to be part and parcel of specific mental conditions are, I believe, perfectly normal ways of coping with a difficult experience of being-in-the-world.[101]

Both autism and schizophrenia represent fascinating conditions. They fascinate neurologists, psychoanalysts, psychologists and the like precisely because it is through the pathology of the mind that many discoveries have been made about how the 'normal' mind works. Even so we must never let the fascination with the pathology obscure the fact that people with autism or schizophrenia are still people. They should be accorded all the dignity and understanding which their humanity demands.

Above all we should not glamorise madness. Much of the 'illness' of mental conditions is caused precisely because the people who have them are having a hard time dealing with their condition. Although there may be ways - that emerge through an understanding of the conditions - that provide opportunities for new 'soft' or cultural treatments (such as getting people who hear voices to positively dialogue with them) drugs, psychotherapeutic and even surgical techniques may be appropriate in some situations.

The challenge in treating any mental illness is twofold. Firstly, we should treat the person as an individual human first and as a 'schizophrenic' second. Secondly, we should use a range of techniques to help that person find their own 'normal' state. The second point is particularly important. Sensitive and empowering therapy can help the individual find their own 'centre', their own form of normality. This does not have to be the normality of the doctor or psychiatrist doing the treatment. Professionals working with mental illness should always be aware that to be 'normal' cannot be narrowly defined. For instance; a patient who is able to deal with his or her audio hallucinations, by externalising these onto a doll (and spending a few hours a day talking with the doll/voice), could be said to be perfectly 'normal'. Their behaviour may not be the same as that of the doctor treating them, but, if the person is calm and able to deal with the full experience of living in a social environment then they can quite legitimately be said to have been healed.

JULIAN VAYNE
## You've Got Everything Now Accept Yourself

'Normal' people exhibit both autistic and schizophrenia behaviours.[102] This is not to say that these conditions are completely culturally dependent, though the line at which treatment or support is offered is subject to cultural conditions. The depths of autistic aloneness or schizophrenic hallucinations are frightening and we should recognise these as situations in which people require a lot of support, understanding and healing. My point is that both schizophrenia and autism represent, I believe, fundamental mental states. We all have them. Some people become trapped in these states, but we all, to a greater or lesser degree, exhibit both these mental relationships with the world. People in numinous states report a feeling that all things are connected - a typical schizophrenic belief. Some people can recall huge amounts of 'trivia', apparently useless and unrelated information - a classic autistic symptom.

I feel that functional parallels exist between the specialisation of the right and left hemisphere of the brain, and the continuum of autism/schizophrenia. Although for some individuals these are undoubtedly 'conditions', for most people both states, both mental views of the world, operate together. Sometimes it is necessary for the mind, as a whole, to be more 'left brain' more 'autistic'. This may be necessary when we learn simple, rule bound or rote knowledge (such as memorising our times tables). At other times a more 'right brain' or schizophrenic approach may be necessary (for gestalt skills, such as riding a bike, or developing the use of metaphorical language). In either case each mental model contains the Derridian trace of its apparent opposite (one might, to paraphrase the description of the Wiccan Goddess say that 'at the heart of the left hemisphere is the right, and at the heart of the right hemisphere lies the left'). After all, in practical terms, there is no point in my memorising my five times table if I cannot use the information in an every-day context. But I may need to strip the information of its practical content, its meaning, in order to effectively rote learn it. After all I'm learning a chant, a string of syllables. However to be encouraged to learn I must be able to see a point, to grasp a reason, moreover I must later be able to apply this knowledge, to 'transfer' it as educationalists say, into another context. I must be able to take my rote learning and use it to accomplish calculations in a range of situations.

## The End of Tears

The cause of both autism and schizophrenia are complex. There is no clear pivotal factor, an exact causal link cannot be established in the case of either condition to viral infections, abnormal foetal development, genetic predisposition or early social environment. Although no single clear candidate for a cause can be found there remains the popular idea that autism (and probably schizophrenia too) has a 'final common pathway'.[103] The rational for this is that autism is a specific constellation of disabilities. Therefore, it seems to follow, that there must be a particular form of damage that occurs to the brain (whatever the cause) the upshot of which is autism. The same logic follows with an analysis of schizophrenia, though since this is a condition that develops later in life (rather than one that prevents usual developmental processes) there tends to be more emphasis on social and environmental factors and less on early developmental damage.

The problem with the 'final common pathway' theory is that it may establish the *mechanism* but not the *situation* of a condition. In one sense this is a general problem of science. We look for the *why* rather than the *whys*. Certainly it may be useful, in terms of treatment, to establish which areas or systems in the brain, when damaged, may lead to autism, but this is not the full story.

Another view would be to imagine autism, as I have done, as a normal part of our mental process. Therefore we can look at autism as being not so much *caused*, instead it is a normal process left *unchecked* by the development of other brain systems. Both schizophrenia and autism are extremes of necessary mental processes that much of our 'normal' mentation is based upon. They are the *solve et coagula* of mental function.

Let's consider the 'final common pathway' in a different context, that of sex. We know that copulation is necessary to reproduction, however we have little understanding of the whole range of other factors that collectively add up to a specific pregnancy. As the archaeologist Timothy Taylor puts it;

> I believe, in every other human community that has ever existed – that women who remain virgin do not become pregnant. Male orgasm is everywhere implicated in the process of human reproduction, but it is everywhere seen as in-sufficient in itself…Many people in the modern world, in both Eastern and Western philosophies, continue to hold the compatible belief that divine intervention is required for the initial implantation of a soul. Speaking for myself, I find the proposition that no spirit is involved in conception unpleasantly atheistic, although I do not deny the physical part that bodies play.[104]

Penetrative, heterosexual sex may be a prerequisite of reproduction but this does not mean that other factors are not necessary too. The 'sex' is the final common pathway but there must be all kinds of exclusions and additions (e.g. one might say 'in order for the woman to fall pregnant the man should not wear a condom', equally the folklore may well be true that 'the recent death of a member of the woman's family is likely to increase her chance of getting pregnant'). Any aspect of human behaviour is *situated* in a web of meanings, some of which may be neurochemical or mechanical, but many of which will be individual and social.

The final common pathway is, I think, misleading, it is the struggling paradigm of western science trying desperately to put an 'equals' sign somewhere in the complexity of human mental life. The oft repeated axiom comes to mind; for every complex problem there is a simple solution - and it's wrong.

## Destination

A stark example of the difficulty in finding the final common pathway comes from the comparative neurochemistry of people with autism and people with schizophrenia. Although it would be more fashionable, at present, to suggest that neurochemical differences have a genetic rather than environmental root, the suggestion that brain chemistry is the final common pathway is a powerful one. The problem with this is that current neurochemical investigations into these disorders have found hazy and, in some respects, quite contradictory evidence. Moreover an explanation, in neurochemical terms only, of autism or schizophrenia might be an example of what the philosopher Daniel Dennett calls pushing the problem back into the 'Cartesian Theatre', the mysterious and, scientifically unapproachable box labelled 'consciousness'.

A number of studies have been done into the neurochemistry of people with both autism and schizophrenia but before we look at these results we need to briefly set neurochemistry in context.

Part of the problem with these studies is that they often rest on animal experiments (with their inevitably dubious results) and on subtle distinctions over what is a core symptom of the illness, and what is a secondary or affective disorder. A more general problem is that neurochemical models are often based on tautological assumptions. So serotonin is the neurotransmitter that makes us feel happy, okay why? Does serotonin carry some sort of happiness quality within itself? Is it that through learning we associate serotonin stimulation with happiness? So why do I feel depressed? Well maybe it's because there is too little serotonin in my brain, why does lack of serotonin make you depressed? Well that's because serotonin makes you happy…and so on.

The circular logic of some neuropharmacology is something that Steven Rose, an expert in memory at the Open University comments on, 'Think of aspirin. It solves the problem of tooth ache but it would be silly to argue that toothache is caused by lack of aspirin.' The situation is reminiscent of Moliere's *Malade Imaginaire* when an examination candidate successfully passes his medical viva. When asked the reason for the narcotic and soporific action of opium 'because it is endowed with narcotic and soporific properties', and, having done no more than re-state the question in the language of the medical discourse, is awarded his qualification.

Certainly I am not denying the value of neurochemical research, however I believe that we must be wary of saying serotonin causes happiness and fixing the emergence of emotions at a chemical level only. There are many processes, some material, some mental, between the chemical messages in the synaptic cleft and our observed or internally experienced states in the human mind. I believe that the feedback system that exists between the neurochemical level and the observed behavioural level should not be underestimated. And this, I think, is clearly demonstrated by the strange case of the inverse findings in autistic and schizophrenia neurochemistry.

## Mysterious Ways

In a significant, but still an overall minority of people with autism who have been tested, higher than average amounts of serotonin have been found in their brain;

The only brain chemical that has clearly been found in abnormal levels in autism is serotonin...It has been discovered that between 30 % and 50% of children with autism have abnormally high levels of serotonin in the blood. Exactly why the levels are high is not known. In children with mental handicap alone, serotonin may also be elevated.[105]

This is observed both as an increase in the number of serotonin receptors in the brain (in post-mortem studies) and as an overall higher concentration in the blood stream.

In similar studies aimed at uncovering a neurochemical basis for schizophrenia a similar pattern emerges, but in this instance it is dopamine that is implicated. Although by no means all patients with autism or schizophrenia share these neurochemical anomalies these observations did suggest some possible directions for drug therapy.

In the case of patients with schizophrenia, neuroleptic (dopamine blocker) drugs have been used, certainly for some people these have proved useful. The psychologist, Tsuang explains, '..the effect of neuroleptics on acute schizophrenia symptoms can be observed only after about two weeks after administration of the drug. It is possible, therefore, that neuroleptics only serve to clear the way, by blocking dopamine receptors, for a second reparative action to take place. What is involved in the second action is still unknown.Neuroleptic drugs are less effective in treating chronic schizophrenia symptoms such as apathy, poverty of ideas, loss of drive or lack of self-care.'

However;
>...increased dopamine response is not important in all schizophrenia patients. In addition, neuroleptic drugs, which block dopamine receptors, are effective only in schizophrenia patients who manifest acute symptoms; delusions or hallucinations.

So neuroleptic drugs serve to alleviate the acute symptoms of schizophrenia ('delusions or hallucinations') but take time to work and do not seem to be able to effect the underlying condition.

An additional part of the schizophrenia puzzle is the effect of high levels of dopamine on 'normal' humans. Amphetamines work by blocking the re-uptake of noradrenaline and dopamine. In large doses amphetamines can generate 'amphetamine psychosis'. This usually consists of paranoia, irritability, perhaps suicidal feelings and, in some cases and at some doses, hallucinations. This lends further weight to the suggestion that somehow dopamine is connected with schizophrenia, however the mystery of the delay in treatment becoming effective, and the fact that only acute symptoms respond to neuroleptic treatment remains.

On the opposite side of the neurochemical coin Tsuang writes that, '...LSD, is also known to produce some features of schizophrenia. The fact that LSD affects the brain receptors of another neurotransmitter, serotonin, led to speculation that a deficiency of serotonin might be involved in schizophrenia.[106] However, serotonin receptors and metabolism were found to be unchanged in the brains of schizophrenic people, rendering this hypothesis untenable. Many studies have investigated other chemicals and enzymes in schizophrenia, but the results are either conflicting of cannot be reproduced.'[107] LSD has been called 'psychotomimetic' – meaning that its effects mimic a psychotic state (although this definition is as dubious as the definition one sees in herbal textbooks of cannabis as 'toxic').[108]

The role of serotonin in autism parallels that of dopamine in schizophrenia. There has certainly been interest in the use of drugs that affect serotonin in the treatment of autism. Fenfluramine has also been used to treat autism. This drug, along with many other dexedrine-like amphetamines, has a 'paradoxical effect'. Rather than cause increased stimulation it has the effect of reducing hyperactive behavior. However the results for these treatments have been inconclusive. Fenfluramine (and related drugs) may have some effect on the more dramatic autistic symptoms, '...reduction in echolalia, perseveration (repetitive behavior) and motor disturbances and an increase in attention and social awareness.'[109]

I have not been able to discover any information detailing apparent time lag (as seen in neuroletpic treatment of schizophrenia) in the effectiveness of fenfluramine treatment. There is however lots of evidence for a significant and pharmacologically odd time lag in the effectiveness of a number of other mind or mood altering drugs. The same two week time lag operates in the case of Prozac and a range of other related drugs. In fact some initial studies on Prozac suggested that some patients found a paradoxical effect after about two weeks. Whereas for most users the drug would start making them feel more relaxed and happy, some people found that they suffered violent outbursts of temper, and even mild 'psychotic symptoms'.

## Dreams made Flesh

I would like to advance a model of drug action and mental processes that may help us make sense of this data. Dopamine might be imagined as the 'ego transmitter', it 'governs' voluntary movement and one's general level of emotional arousal.[110] Dopamine might be considered the 'yang' of the neurochemical continuum, it is the 'left brain' neurotransmitter.

Serotonin is the 'Other' transmitter, it governs sleep and alterations within the serotonin system that can lead to changes in perception of time and environment.[111] Serotonin is the 'yin' in our system, the 'right brain' chemical messenger.

I am keenly aware at this point that friends of mine who are neurologists and pharmacologists will be bemoaning my quasi-scientific generalisations. However as I have said in order to explore the actions of drugs a barefoot model of their relationships may be useful.[112] For example, if we look at the role of serotonin and dopamine in the cases of autism and schizophrenia we find a situation that seems to fly in the face of my broad generalisation. Autism is, quintessentially a condition of 'Self'. Held back by the imaginative discontinuity, the mind of the autistic person only knows itself. It would therefore seem logical that we should see dopamine implicated in this condition – yet it is the 'opposite' neurotransmitter that seems to have a role, in at least the more serious forms of the illness.

Equally with the terrifying conspiracies and hallucinations of schizophrenia, one would assume that people with severe symptoms would show greater than normal levels of serotonin in their brains. This would create a neat link between the role of LSD as a serotonin mimic and it's 'psychotomimetic' effect.[113]

In both cases the results are quite counter-intuitive, and certainly seem opposed to the broad model of dopamine related to 'Self', serotonin related to 'Other' that I have proposed. However I believe that there are two important pieces of information that can help us to unravel the puzzle.

The first is the time delay that occurs in treatment with neuroleptic drugs (and, I suspect, is paralleled with Fenfluramine). This delayed action is certainly experienced by people being treated with anti-depressants that modify neurotransmitter function.

The second is the fact that these treatments (whatever neurochemical system is being altered) only work in the most severe of cases or on the most dramatic of symptoms. The underlying condition remains unchecked.

## A Secret Life

My belief that autism and schizophrenia are a functional duality, serves to show one of the most important points when it comes to understanding drugs. The current fashion, when exploring the action of drugs on the mind, is to build models from the ground up, taking as read that the mind is a 'virtual machine' (as the materialist philosopher Daniel Dennet puts it) that runs like a computer program upon the hardware of the neurochemical and neurological systems. Although I am not denying the role of neurochemistry and anatomy on the mind I think that the process is certainly a two-way street. In short, the contents of the mind structure the relationship with the neurochemical situation in the brain just as much as the neurochemical state of the brain effects the mental state.

For example: the overproduction of dopamine in the brain chemistry of some schizophrenic people may not be the cause of their schizophrenia, rather it may be a result. It could be that the mind of the schizophrenic person attempts to protect and maintain a sense of Self in the face of a SuperReal universe (certainly the behaviours of many schizophrenia people, such as not eating because 'the conspiracy is out to poison them', is a perfectly logical way trying to preserve the Self under extraordinary conditions). The production of dopamine may well be the neurochemical expression of the schizophrenic mind trying to force a coherence in an incoherent, hallucination filled world.

Likewise the prevalence of serotonin in autistic individuals may be the neurochemical expression of the mind trying to create relationship in a world where relationships do not exist.

To put it simply; the chemical changes in our brains both *underlie and express* what we think. In autism and schizophrenia, using serotonin and dopamine agonists respectively may alleviate some symptoms but I think that these symptoms are due not so much to the neurochemical effects of these chemicals, as they are to do with quieting minds that are desperately seeking a way out of their predicament. This view is supported by the fact that both treatments only address the most dramatic symptoms but do not seem to affect the underlying condition.

If this analysis is born out by research it would not be the first time the blame has been pinned on the wrong candidate in medical research. It was initially assumed that cholesterol was the cause of some heart attacks. Now it is recognised that, although some forms of cholesterol do increase the chances of heart attacks, cholesterol is also secreted by the body *after* a heart attack as part of the healing process. The high levels of cholesterol initially found in the bloodstream of heart attack victims led to the assumption that cholesterol was the *cause* and not the *outcome* of the condition.

## Violently Happy

On a day to day basis all sorts of neuropharmacological intervention is used in the treatment of mental illness. In practice much of this boils down to giving sedatives, antidotes to their side-effects, antidepressants and so forth.[114] Using a single drug is unlikely to repair any organic problem or provide a complete remedial treatment for behavioural difficulties. Indeed pharmacologists and others are quite aware of 'using a sledgehammer to crack a nut' that drug intervention can imply.[115] One problem with many of these drugs is simply that they become tremendously popular, in part due to marketing and in part due to our culture's desire to pop a pill and get well. The phenomenal rise of drugs such as Ritalin (an amphetamine used to treat 'attention deficit disorder' – hyperactivity – in children) and anti-depressants like Prozac are witness to this.

It is certainly understandable, given the sorrow that mental illness can cause, that our society should eagerly grasp at even the most primitive of straws. So what else can we do? I think that in drug therapy it would seem advantageous to consider two important points which are exemplified by the conditions autism and schizophrenia. One, it is useful to understand the 'paradoxical effect' that drugs can have, and two, to appreciate that *the effect of a drug is perceived by the mind*.

We are used to the paradox where extracts are taken from snake venom to produce an antidote to snake bite. We are used to the idea that inoculations protect us from disease precisely because they expose us to a weak form of a virus. What we are less familiar with is the paradoxical role of drugs. Ritalin, mentioned above, is speed, yet it calms down children with hyperactivity. Dopamine function is not itself associated with hallucinations and mental confusion, yet it appears as a common factor in some cases of acute schizophrenia.

We are also used to drugs having an effect on the body but we tend to neglect the effect of drugs on the mind, and certainly the effect of the mind on the perception of drug experience. This information is vitally important when we come to consider mental illness. After all, tranquillisers may stop a mentally ill patient from wandering aimlessly around but I do not feel that they can really be said to have helped his or her mental state as a whole.

We should remember that a drug is not just a chemical that changes the flow of neurotransmitters across the synaptic cleft – a drug is also (and, I believe, first and foremost) an experience. The way an individual person responds to a drug depends as much on how that person conceptualises the experience as any preconceived ideas of what system a given chemical stimulates or depresses. We do not simply *have* neurochemical effects, but we also give those effects *meaning* through our mental *interpretation* of the drug experience.

The work of Freud is important when we look at the symptoms of mental illness. Freud's development of psychoanalysis rests upon the notion that symptoms displayed within mental illness represent a self-protective mechanism within the mind. Moreover each symptom can provide the therapist with a road inward to assist in the 'abreaction' (i.e. the release of repressed emotional trauma from the unconscious) or curing of the illness. Given Freud's model we could read the extreme hallucinations of schizophrenia as the brain trying to make sense of the world through visual fantasy. Equally the excess of dopamine, in schizophrenic people with acute symptoms, supports the interpretation that these symptoms represent an attempt by the mind to seek meaningful coherence. Though a condition such as schizophrenia may have organic factors (neural damage, genetic predisposition), we need to use the symptoms to gain a road in to the healing process. Learning to dialogue with one's 'voices' isn't only a stop-gap measure in the treatment of schizophrenia, it is actually a healing process.

So too in the case of autism, obsessive rituals are the autistic person's way of keeping their world together. We shouldn't seek to treat these people with drugs that only remove these behaviours. If mental illness is treated as a solely organic event, not only are we likely to be treating only the symptoms and not effecting a cure, but we are also likely to be damaging the very processes that the mind can use to heal, or at least cope with, the illness itself.

## When I Walk Through the Land of Fear

If, for instance, serotonin overproduction by some autistic people, is a symptom of their mind fighting for release, it would seem reasonable to attempt to help the body's own system rather than seek to oppose it pharmacologically. Interestingly there is a drug that effects serotonin re-uptake that, in many people's experience, provides just the sort of experiences of relaxation, communication and heightened sense of imagination and relationship that autistic people lack. That drug is MDMA.

The idea of using MDMA in the treatment of autism has been suggested before, most notably by Dr Morris A. Lipton (who testified at the MDMA Scheduling Hearings in the USA); 'Childhood autism is an essentially untreatable condition in which the child is unable to relate to significant people in his environment. MDMA might be tried with such children, partly because the reported effects of enhancing communication among adults might be helpful in autism.'

As far as I am aware this type of therapy has never been tried. LSD does certainly give some access to the world akin to the hallucinations that plague the schizophrenic (and indeed it, and psilocybin have been used in therapeutic contexts). Perhaps other drugs that effect the dopamine system might be used to help the schizophrenic person to develop a coherent sense of Self. In any case the hallucinations of schizophrenia are seen not as 'the enemy' but rather as a feature of the condition (much as a runny nose is one sign of having a cold). Careful use of drug therapy might well seek to engage and work with schizophrenic hallucinations (perhaps by combining LSD and psychotherapy) rather than simply turn them off. As is the case with 'flu, drying up one's runny nose does not treat the underlying condition, and may even serve to prolong the course of the illness.

Whether such therapies as applied pharmacology alone would work is, I believe, doubtful. Indeed the delay in the effectiveness of neuroleptic treatment of schizophrenia may point the way. If we use our 'set a thief to catch a thief' logic then it rests as much on how the patient *experiences* the drug induced change as it does on neurochemical action itself. I believe that the reduction in symptoms in neuroleptic therapy is due to the reduction in the sense of paranoia that schizophrenia people understandably experience. The time lag is due to the mind realising that it is itself less stressed. What we are witnessing is not a delayed pharmacological reaction as much as a change in the patient's own mental orientation towards their own experiences. The schizophrenic on neuroleptics may experience fewer hallucinations and would certainly be less nervous of them. However the underlying condition, the lack of a separate, autistic 'I', is still there.

To produce a more long-term solution support therapies are necessary. This is painfully obvious for anyone who is on Prozac (which may make you feel happier in general terms) who has been offered a stopgap pharmacological solution, where a blend of drug treatment, counselling, and social assistance might have been more useful.

If we seek to use, for instance, MDMA to help people with autism this must be linked to supportive therapies. The brain may require drugs to change its state but the effect of these drugs must be supported and made meaningful in terms of the mind's experience.

Using the above interpretation of this pairing of mental illnesses and neurochemical data, we might suggest the following model. This model is based on a reading of schizophrenia but could certainly be adapted to elucidate autism also.

Organic illness leads to unconscious illness, an inability to 'play' between autistic and schizophrenic states of being. This in turn generates conscious symptoms (E.g. poverty of ideas, lassitude, then acute symptoms (hallucinations), and finally panic (since these symptoms are those of 'madness'). Extreme symptoms lead to changes in neurochemical production within the brain, which is an attempt at a reparative action. This process can also be displayed in behaviour which, though 'mad' can be interpreted as an intelligent attempt at seeking mental coherence and wellbeing.

Effective treatment lies not in simply stopping the mind of the sufferer being 'locked' at one or other extreme of the autistic-schizophrenic scale (which only means reduction of acute symptoms). Instead it means assisting the individual to develop a flexible but stable sense of 'I'.

So although conditions such as schizophrenia, in part, may be an organic illness, the symptoms need to be treated as much as mental and social events as well as an organic dysfunction.

## Inbetweener

As we have set the conditions of autism and schizophrenia within a broader context, to include both neurochemical *and* mental factors, let us contextualise the medical science that seeks to cure or control mental illness.

Historically most neurology stands firmly in the tradition of materialism. That is the belief that anything, the world as a whole and specifically the mind, can be explained by the scientific investigation of known physical laws. The logic runs that, at least in principle, the mind and all its contents can, at some future time, be explained as being caused by the interaction of neurones, chemicals, electrical impulses and, eventually, the laws of physics. Aside from the problems that modern physics presents for materialism (even the most fundamental particles in the universe are taking on a more and more ghostly appearance with the advent of quantum mechanics) the materialist position is ultimately a *philosophical* one.

An opposing view to materialism is that postulated by Descartes, namely *dualism* or more accurately, *interactionalism*. Descartes' theories have been the whipping boy for materialism, and its scions of behaviourism, cognitive science and neurology. This position is taken up by the philosopher Daniel Dennett in *Consciousness Explained*, 'The idea of mind as distinct in this way from the brain, composed not of ordinary matter but of some other, special kind of stuff, is *dualism*, and it is deservedly in disrepute today.'[116]

The assertions of materialist science, in its various incarnations, bring it up against many philosophical problems. Many of these questions have a direct impact on the nature and implications of practical research and the interpretation of data. For instance; is it philosophically possible for the mind to 'know itself'? Would it ever be meaningful to talk (using presumably one's mind to frame the thoughts) about understanding how the mind itself builds the ideas that it is speaking? The problem becomes a knotted circle. Rather than acknowledging any limit to scientific knowledge, even a limit created by our need to *interpret* scientific ideas, neurology is seeking its own holy grail: the grand unified theory of the mind.

But there are voices raised against the theoretical possibility of attaining this neurological holy grail. Philosophers such as Colin McGinn argue that we cannot have a full account of how the brain works simply because we will be experiencing that information through the brain itself.[117] To put the problem another way; if the brain were so simple we could understand it, then we'd be so stupid that we couldn't!

Today, a major player in the materialist discourses of science is the study of artificial intelligence and computers. Neurology is increasingly being informed by computer studies and technological developments. Academic and scientist, Colin Blakemore writes:

> In this century the metaphors [for how the brain works] have shifted again and again, with each new leap in technology. The brain was 'an enchanted loom', a telephone exchange, a hologram or a chemical plant. But the most forceful and in some ways frightening metaphor is that of the computer. A computer, in the broadest sense, is an engine of calculation, a device for processing information according to a program – a set of formal instructions. With such a compliant definition as this, the brain is not simply *like* a computer; it *is* a computer.[118]

Artificial intelligence (AI) has to grapple with the same big questions as neurology, since both are attempting to create physical models (computer systems or electro-chemical sequences) of known mathematical systems that will, presumably spontaneously, generate a mind. The basic premise of neurology - that mind emerges out of a complex interaction of firing synapses - can easily be translated into the metaphor of binary systems in computers. A brain cell according to these theories is, in a simplistic but essentially identical way, a switch. The idea that the mind is the 'software' to the binary zeros and ones of the brain's 'hardware', is an eagerly accepted analogy. Since, if the analogy holds true, we might really be able to build a mind out of lots of little switches – to create an artificial intelligence. AI has been a strong growth area in modern science. There were initially high hopes, buoyed up in part by significant military funding, though to date nothing approaching an artificial intelligence has been built.[119]

Of course computers are capable of amazing feats of 'autistic' processing power. Famously this is how IBM's system 'Deep Blue' beat chess grandmaster Gary Kasparov in May 1997. Although Kasparov complained that it was as though the machine 'knew what he was thinking', Deep Blue is far from a true AI system.[120] What it does demonstrate is the vast developments of processing capacity that have occurred in recent years. Who can say what the technological outcome of the AI project will be? Perhaps one day we may well be able to create something resembling the 'minds' in Iain M Banks' science fiction novels.[121] But the problem of creating a mind that we, as humans, would recognise as another mind (and be able to communicate with), rests as much with overcoming philosophical problems as it does technical ones.

I would not deny the use and value of computer systems, or indeed of examining computational models of the mind. My disagreement is with the notion of the simple causal equivalence of the models being proposed. I believe that the mind is about *interpretation* and the materialist vision is only one interpretation of the world. It is not an absolute 'objective' truth. In terms of AI this problem is compounded by seeing *similarity* or *relationship* as *identity*. To reiterate what Blakemores' claim, '…the brain is not simply *like* a computer; it *is* a computer.'

Of course the metaphor of mind and computer may be useful, may be an interesting *interpretation*. Certainly there are scientists who use computers to model mental behaviour without believing that the mind *is* a computer. One of the most notable is Gerald Edelman, Nobel Prize winner and neurologist, who remarked, 'Whatever their interest or usefulness, neural networks are not adequate models or analogues of brain structures.'[122]

Models which liken the mind to a computer were certainly being used in the 1960s, during the exploration of LSD. Both Lilly and Leary use language which describes the mind in terms of 'biocomputers' and 'circuits of contelligence'. Many writers about drug experience are themselves very excited about the developments in neurology and AI. Even something of the cultural excitement of being at a 'new frontier' in the study of the mind slips between disciplines. Writer Jay Steven takes up this point in his excellent history of LSD and psychedelic culture in his book *Storming Heaven*:

> The neuroconsciousness frontier, circa 1983, reminded me a lot of the psychedelic movement, circa 1962...There was the same quality of excitement, the same mix of therapeutic and metaphysical interests, the same cautious optimism.[123]

Although the vision of neurology persists and there are many excellent research projects currently being undertaken, there is still a strong emphasis on materialist philosophy in these sciences. The ritual of banishing the 'ghost from the machine' seeks to replace it with admittedly complex, but essentially knowable, content. This project is opposed to the philosophies that are inherent in a number of other disciplines. This included psychoanalysis and much psychology which proposes an 'unconscious' mind, a part of experience which is simultaneously responsible for a number of our behaviours but which, by definition, cannot be conscious. Although in therapy one aim is to make unconscious material available to conscious scrutiny, we cannot do this with the whole of the unconscious mind simultaneously. Not to have an unconscious mind, according to psychoanalysis, is not to be human. Is it philosophically possible to consciously understand and build an unconscious mind?

If we are to understand the mind we must make deliberate provision for the possibility that some parts of it may be, as Wittgenstein puts it 'unspeakable'. In practical terms we must be willing to acknowledge the possibility that we simply do not and may not be able to know everything. A grand unified theory of consciousness, physics or indeed of everything, is a cultural monolith that the human process of transgression will never allow to remain in place. As a friend pointed out to me 'okay so let's say we get a unified theory of everything, will it be able to explain whether I like the theory or not?'

## States of Mind

What would a broader understanding of the mind, and drug experience in particular look like? I believe that a more well-rounded approach to drug experience needs to include 'set, setting and substance'. Substance is the drug, or rather the drug experienced through the body. This means both the physical material of the drug (the dosage and its chemical constituents) and the physical tolerances and state of the body. The body of the individual must be thought of in the broadest sense. For example what food has been eaten in the last few hours will effect how a given drug operates. Gender, genetics, general level of fitness, the presence of particular diseases or stresses are all factors.

We could of course go on pursuing the concept of 'the body' in the set, setting, substance triad until we realise that subtle factors such as time of the day or season will have physiological effects upon the individual organism.[124] As well as dosage and the state of the physical body itself, the manner of absorption of the drug is also important. It is in the context of the preferred route of administration that we can see how the set, setting and substance concepts fuse. For example heroin used intravenously is more than simply a fast and effective means of administration. It has sociological and cultural (external - setting) and psychic and personal (internal - set) meanings.[125] Although the use of intravenous techniques is certainly the most 'loaded' with cultural and symbolic significance in our culture, other methods of preparation and administration also have a psychic as well as pragmatic meaning.

For some drugs experience shows that the route of administration makes few differences. For instance, MDMA injected will 'come on' faster than that swallowed, but intravenous use does not seem to increase the subjective high. This is quite different from cocaine, which, subjectively, can produce a much more powerful rush when injected which renders it a very different drug experience to that derived from snorting.[126]

Neurochemistry and pharmacology must become interdisciplinary studies, drawing on other areas of enquiry that may well be at odds with a materialist philosophy of the world. Drug experience is a fusion of set, setting and substance, it is an *experience* which can usefully be analysed at a number of levels.

## Are you Experienced?

Our exploration of drugs in neurochemical and pharmacological terms demonstrates many of the same features of drug experience that I identified in the first chapter. Namely that we must speak of drugs as experience. That although we can make broad generalisations about the effect of certain chemicals, we must always be open to individual variations, and realise that the individual experience (the set and setting) can be profoundly different.

Although in the sections that follow I will generalise about the effect of particular drugs, I am keenly aware of the variation in actual drug experience. If nothing else most drugs have a paradoxical nature. Just the right amount of digitalis will even out an irregular heat beat, too much and it will cause a heart attack. Camphor, in small doses is an anti-convulsant. In larger doses it will cause convulsions. Barbiturates will make most people sleepy but will stimulate a catatonic schizophrenic person into action…and so forth.

When we speak of the reason for say, MDMA making us social and happy as being that it causes a change in serotonin re-uptake, we must be aware that what we are saying is not a complete explanation. Certainly, at the neurochemical level this is the effect, but at the level of mental experience it is just as meaningful to say that we are happy because MDMA blurs interpersonal boundaries.

The models of mind proposed by occultism or its daughter sciences (e.g. psychoanalysis and psychology) are just as useful as the models generated by neuropharmacology. Materialists such as Daniel Dennett and the host of cognitive scientists contend that a real understanding of the mind will be made when we link mental states back to chemical changes in the brain. I think that this is only half the story and that we must also take account of the way the mind *understands* the changes that are taking place within the brain.[127] Ultimately we need to understand much of the action of a given drug from a social and psychic perspective. We are not just a collection of chemicals, we are thinking, feeling selves. To make drug experience meaningful we have to have a psychic 'human scale' description as well as a neurochemical analysis. For instance, heroin addicts are not only addicts because endorphins are under-produced in their neurochemistry. They are addicts because of social, psychological, economic and other factors. In the climate of science today one might add 'they are heroin addicts because of their genes'. But, as geneticists themselves will generally admit 'for' is the most dangerous word in the vocabulary of genetics. There may be genetic factors that make heroin addition more likely, but that is quite different from saying that there is a gene for heroin addiction.[128]

(I would not wish to tar all neurologists with the same brush. Certainly writers such as Antionio Damasio do point out that '…reducing depression to a statement about the availability of serotonin or norepinephrine…is unacceptabily rude.' Although Damasio, along with most of his colleagues still insists on emphasising the 'bottom up' process of brain function giving rise to mental function.)[129]

We do not simply *have* experiences, be they of madness or intoxication, we are also engaged in the ongoing process of *making sense* of them. Recognising the role of the mind in research on the brain would be a powerful step for biological science to take.

## Placebo

As we leave the realm of neurology and take our examination of drugs into a wider arena, it is worth pausing a moment to consider an explicit example of the power of the mind.

The placebo effect is a great example of the 'bootstrapping' process of the mind, where the mind can effect itself, and systems of the body that we normally imagine as being outside of our control. Simply by telling someone (in a convincing enough way) that an inert substance is a powerful drug, can give rise to very significant 'drug-like' effects.

In one study subjects who were experiencing pain were given three types of painkillers. These ranged from aspirin, through a stronger pain killer, to morphine. Patients were asked, on a scale or one to three (three being high) to rate the effectiveness of the pain killing drugs. As might be expected, although individuals did vary in their reactions, the majority of people rated aspirin as one, the next drug as two and morphine as three.

Trials were then conducted using placebo pills, variously described as being aspirin, a medium strength painkiller and morphine. In these cases people who received the placebo which claimed to be morphine rated it as 2.3, higher than the real medium-strength painkiller. This high rating serves to demonstrate how powerful the placebo effect is. It also serves to underline that the mind can massively influence the body (if we imagine a neurologically-centred view of humans where pain is changes in neurochemistry). Moreover it supports the assertion that a drug is primarily an experience (rather than a substance). The 'ritual', or set and setting influences, surrounding the use of the placebo was that it contained morphine, and that morphine is a powerful painkilling drug. In just the same way therapy with drugs, to be effective, should seek to contextualise the experience in terms that support the therapeutic aim. So rather than just doling out Prozac and tricyclic antidepressants as a chemical solution, drug users (be they patients, health care workers or shamanic healers) must attempt to use the fact that the mind, and its relationship to the drug experience, is an important factor in the effectiveness of the treatment.

The effect of a given drug is also affected by memory, both of previous drug experiences and of similar states of consciousness. The first time I took LSD I had a very easy and positive trip (despite an inadvertently high dose). In part I think this was because I had spent years studying and practising ritual magic, meditation and mental skills. I was aware that, though the acid experience was new, it was similar to, yet different from the states that I had explored using other methods of changing consciousness. My memory of other 'altered states' of consciousness influenced and helped me deal with the LSD experience.

Although I have never experienced anything that might be called an LSD 'flashback' I have had similar 'memory-driven' experiences with MDMA. I remember that for up to two weeks after taking my first pill in a club, the sound of repetitive dance music would awaken a subtle but definite feeling of 'coming up'. In this case memory itself, and associations between ecstasy and dance music, was the placebo.

It would be interesting to know whether familiarity with the drug enhances the placebo effect, or whether because you know how the drug should feel the substitution of the active chemical with a placebo would be more obvious. I suspect that this is something of degrees, in that if you give somebody enough supportive environmental evidence (for example, dance music, a relaxed atmosphere, the story that 'these pills are really subtle but actually quite strong') it would be possible to generate some significant effect even in somebody who is used to taking ecstasy. Writer Nicholas Saunders reports that;

> A trial using male actors found that LSD subjects experienced maximum loss of control after 30 minutes, and this declined gradually. 'After two hours, subjects reported feelings of having acquired new meanings and a more prominent general feeling of disinhibition.' The researchers found that those who had taken placebos experienced similar types of symptoms at 2, 5 and 8 hours after ingestion, although the symptoms varied from strong to very weak.
>
> With marijuana, some placebos were made by extracting varying amounts of the active ingredient THC. The symptoms reported by most subjects were consistent with strength, but the unexpected result was that chronic users felt stronger reactions from the placebo.

Similar effects have also been found with regard to cocaine.[130] There is a strange twist within the placebo effect, whereby, in the case of hashish

'Marijuana users probably develop a similar increase in sensitivity – what is sometimes called "reverse tolerance"- to marijuana's effects.'[131] This type of sensitisation is a well documented medical phenomena, paralleled in some respects by the practice of immunisation. Once again the drug experience is paradoxical and we are called to admit the relationship of the Self to the chemical experience within the pharmacological description of what is happening.

Personally, I know that during one of the most powerful LSD experiences I (and my partner) started to 'come up' within 10 minutes, far too short a time (according to mechanistic neurochemistry) to allow the drug to have started to have any effect. But I know what I felt. Set, setting and substance had combined together with a powerful synergy. In a literal sense, we were tripping before the drug started to work.[132]

The power of the placebo is such that it can affect even the most experienced drug user. Alexander Shulgin describes how he had to undergo an emergency operation during the war. Before the operation he was given a glass of orange juice with a white powder at the bottom. He was immediately sent unconscious by the mixture which afterwards he was told was nothing more than orange juice and sugar.[133]

The placebo effect is not simply about illusion, since its effects can be so physical, in terms of functions such as pain control, rate of blood loss in haemorrhaging, dilation of pupils and so on. A placebo (i.e. set and setting without significant substance) can affect not only what we normally think of as having some measure of control over (i.e. our experience of how we feel), but it can also affect processes that we normally consider to be automatic, unconscious and quite separate from what we think of as 'ourselves'.

## Head like a Hole

When we speak of the mind, we do tend to equate this with the brain, what occultist Pete Carroll calls the 'two and a half pounds of electrified fat inside our skulls'. Our tendency is to locate the mind 'within' the brain, but this location is as much cultural as it is anatomical. I know that 'I' have a unitary sense of being but in reality my body is a complex community of cells. This includes the virtually independent flora and fauna of my gut, the near-independent mitochondria cells in my body, indeed it includes my sperm cells that are capable of moving out from my body to help create a new human being.

The human mind is contained not only within the chemical interactions taking place within my skull, but also in a continuous web of sensations, cultural meanings, subtle senses (what writer Peter Redgrove calls the 'dark senses')[134] such as my subliminal awareness of barometric pressure, electro-magnetic fields, pheromone scents, and so forth. For this reason it is hardly surprising that setting has such an important effect on any drug that I might take; setting is one aspect of who 'I' am.

The idea that 'I' am behind my eyes is as much due to the visual orientation of our society as it is because 'I' live, in some objective way, 'inside' the organ in my head. After all, the mind itself does not have an exact location. Although we may look at neuropathologies (such as those examined by clinician and writer Oliver Sacks) and suggest that damage to certain parts of the brain causes damage to some functions of the mind, the mind itself is a concept that can be internalised (or indeed externalised) in many different ways. Oriental cultures and some Native American peoples locate the self in the stomach or near the navel.

In fact there are some interesting accounts of neurological damage (usually accompanied by psychological trauma) that demonstrate quite clearly how our location of self is really quite arbitrary. There is an account of a World War I soldier who, after being hit by a shell, woke up to find 'himself' floating in the corner of the infirmary, looking down on his body. In this account he gradually returned to a conception of himself as within his skull as he recovered. But during his experience he conceptualised all his sensory experience as being from his new perspective. The power of the mind to shift our apparent location of perception is shown by near death experiences (and other out of body states) where the body is seen as if from outside.

The changes in the mind, whether they are brought about through techniques such as biofeedback, visualisation, the placebo effect or whatever, arise from our imaginative faculties. In just the same way we can imagine the world outside our bodies. When a drug gives us the experience of dislocation (in the way that ketamine does) we should remember that this is not only a chemical experience, it is also an imaginative mental one. The experience of flying when one takes datura represents a real change in one's imagined location of mind. You could call it a 'chemical experience' or 'drug induced hallucination' but how true is it that you live 'behind' your eyes, and how useful is it to explain any complex experience (such as love or grief) as the action of chemicals alone?

## Life, Love and Unity

The very fact that we experience ourselves (albeit located 'in' our skulls) surrounded by a continuous flow of sensory and innerworld experience (or set and setting) is a testament to the power of human imagination. This ability to imagine, to locate a personal sense of self in the world is what makes learning (as a group or as an individual) possible.

The ability to imagine is essential to learning, even though imagination has been castigated in the materialist world; 'At present we are completely unequipped to think about the subjective character of experience without relying on the imagination – without taking up the point of view of the experimental subject.'[135]

But the point is that imagination is essential to being. People with autism are unable to grasp the full use of the imagination. This does not mean that autistic people cannot learn. However, they have a severely curtailed repertoire of methods for learning since they have not passed the imaginative discontinuity. A person with autism, like the left hemisphere of the brain, learns in isolated sequence.

The autistic[136] speech of a young child (as the psychologist Piaget calls it) is the 'speech for itself' but this is undifferentiated from speech outside of the child (which comes from friends, parents etc.), it is not yet true communication between Self and Other. We might think of rote learning and rule bounded systems (such as chess, geometry or names and dates history) as being 'autistic' in that they represent information dealt with in the sort of sequential bits that we make computers process. Indeed if processing sequential bits were all a human mind (including one that is diagnosed as 'autistic') could do then the arguments from proponents of artificial intelligence would be more satisfying. But it is the imagination that firmly positions us in the world of social experience and meaningful knowledge (rather than the amazing but obtuse knowledge of the autistic person). It is imagination that turns the child's autistic speech into true communication.

Yet this is not to deny the value of sequential learning or 'autistic' thought, it is a vital part of a whole process. Schizophrenia shows us what happens when the imaginative, gestalt loving 'right hemisphere' system gets out of balance. The self becomes lost in the incoming sensory data. Unable to discriminate between the personal and the general, the 'meant for me' and the general hubbub of the world, everything becomes intense, meaningful and, usually, frightening.

I believe that we as humans must straddle the boundary between the autistic/sequential and schizophrenic/gestalt modes of perception. If we enter the realm of autism (be it through drug experience or the experience of becoming a rationalist scientist) we must be able to make our knowledge meaningful to those people around us. If we project ourselves outward into the realm of schizophrenia (perhaps through art or mysticism) we must be able to return to the sequential world of spoken language and linear time.

## What the World is Waiting For

It is not simply for the chemical effect that we use drugs to make changes in our social world. Rather it is because drugs help us to learn by giving us the license and the support to enter new relationships (to move through the 'zone of proximal development'). As a liminal experience a drug is both a *thing* and a *feeling*, something which throws into relief the everyday negotiations between our schizophrenic and autistic modes of being.

Drinking champagne is much more than simply absorbing alcohol, it is a 'multivocal' symbol.[137] Our use of drugs in seduction, grief, relaxation and celebration (whether it be wine, cannabis or peyote) is the social expression of the drive that spurs the shaman to traffic with the dangerous experiences of datura or henbane intoxication.

In many cultures, and throughout much of history, drugs have been used to mark the transition between social states. In western culture the ubiquitous drug alcohol is used to 'wet the babies head' as it is born, later the child may undergo the little formalised event of getting drunk at an adolescent party. If the individual is a Christian, wine will serve as the medium for divine grace in its religious life. Marriage bonds are toasted and, in time, a tipple at the wake will be required to send the individual into the world of the ancestors.

In political terms tea parties (whether of the British Women's Institute or of the Boston variety) may become the centres for political action. We might speak of the drunken mob of rioters but there is no direct causal link alcohol=riots any more than there is a gene for civil disobedience, or that tea literally brews revolution. Rather the drug gives us permission to change, it is the focal meeting place of minds, and is itself symbolic of the autopoietic transgression we decide upon.

The drug as the catalyst for social change, is synergistic with our neurochemistry and our cultural and social expectations. The drugs do not do the job of affecting change, our imaginative ability, and our paradoxical skill of comprehending the world as sequential and yet continuous experience, does that. So however much we plumb the neurochemical reactions of chemicals we should always remember that drugs are primarily, like sexuality and beauty, in the mind.

Drugs are the fruits from the tree of knowledge. They can certainly be used to enslave but that is no reason to reject them. Art can be turned towards small-minded propaganda purposes but this does not mean that art is bad. Drugs remind us to be careful about setting apparently firm boundaries between Self and Other. They remind us that even though we think we know something of how the brain works, we do so only through the mind itself. They show us how we can change our perceptions, our location and concept of self. They can be a strong medicine, capable of breaking people out of entrenched complexes and ways of being. But they warn us to be careful. For we must learn to make the shamanic return from the drug state and realise that what we seek to accomplish with the transgression of drug use is up to us.

# Movements of a Visionary: drugs and the occult

### Take Me to the Other Side

In this section I will examine, in more general terms, the power and value of drug experience, and set the drug experience within a more directly esoteric context.

I believe that drugs can be used in a transformative or 'self actualising' way. This does not only include the type of self transformation that we are familiar with from therapy and counselling (though these healing techniques should not be under valued) but also transformations of a more esoteric type. Drugs can allow us to transgress the limitations and structures of our bodies, drugs can allow us access to a variety of invisible worlds, drugs can confer special abilities and insights.

I do not propose to give a scientific analysis of, nor support for my more 'occult' claims. What I state in the following pages has been born out of my own experience and can be supported through ethnographic data. I will begin by examining some of the basic concepts that drug experience challenges: dualities such as Self/Other and Law/Chaos as well as refining the idea of transgression by considering its philosophical implications and the esoteric traditions in which it appears.

Perhaps some of the more outlandish experiences and abilities that are reported by drug users are indeed 'all in the mind'. The question though remains: what are the limits of our minds?

## Us and Them

We make differences between Self and Other, and between inner sensations and external conditions.

What we choose to include as 'I' can be radically different from person to person and culture to culture. Thus the idea that I own my body, and therefore have the right to determine when it will cease to function (since I believe that voluntary euthanasia is morally acceptable) is quite opposed to a Catholic Christian view. In the view of those opposed to abortion or suicide 'I' do not own my body. The location for decisions concerning it is located outside of my physical being (with God, or the State, or the Law).

As another example: I find it perfectly normal to swallow my own saliva, but most people would be repulsed by the idea of drinking a glass of spittle (even if it was their own). Thus the boundary of Self/not-Self, or the locus for our intentionality is a moveable feast.

The system that we develop of making differences, of defining the boundaries of 'Self' and 'Other' is fundamentally mutable. The mutability of this system is what we call learning. For example when I first tried to use a mouse on a computer I found the whole process ridiculously difficult. I'd find, as thousands of other computer users do, that my desk simply wasn't big enough! The arrow pointer would be hard to the left of the screen but I'd run out of physical space to track the mouse! Once I was shown how it is possible to lift the mouse (thus keeping the pointer in the same location, but allowing me to re-position the mouse on the desk so that the ball could continue to track) I began to understand how to use the device. This is a simple example of learning. At first I was able to understand the basic principles of the mouse. The arrow as a virtual pointer on the screen, and certain areas of the screen designated as 'buttons', 'windows' etc. This much made sense, but I was unable to extend my 'self' into the pointer since I was limited by my understanding of how to physically manipulate the mouse. I learnt the technique, so that now I never even notice 'running off the desk' when I use the mouse. The whole effect is, as far as any tool can be that I still register as 'separate' from my Self, seamless.[138]

Generally we do not perceive tools as entirely seamless parts of ourselves, however in order to develop virtuoso guitar playing, painting or cricket, the tool must become, quite literally, part of the body. A car driver extends her sense of body space, in order to drive safely, to include the surrounding cage of metal. Not only can the physical shape of the body change (as in the case of the car driver being unconsciously aware of the size of the car) but the functions of the body can change too. Thus for the accomplished piano player it becomes meaningless to ask whether the music is made by the piano or by the pianist. Equally the jet pilot, using infra-red goggles and travelling faster than sound has a body with very specially adapted abilities.

This ability to learn to locate the 'body' (that is the physical extent of where 'I' have voluntary control) outwards, to re-locate the sense of Self, is exactly the same ability whether it appears as a seamless link between the fencer and her sword, the cultural perception that 'I' live in my skull, or out-of-body-experiences where the self is located floating above the operating table.

## And Here I Stand

'I' am a fiction, my continuity of consciousness is really full of gaps. Yet my history seems pretty much seamless. I know that every night I loose consciousness of myself and come round hours later without any sense that I have 'lost time'. I am not composed of the same cells that I was made of when I was born, my memory is continuously being re-written, my opinions and experiences change, my sense of my body (as shown above) changes - and yet I am still 'I'.

When we consider the power of drug experiences and learning in general to *change* our sense of Self, to make us 'different', we must also recognise the simultaneous truth of our sense of *self continuity*. Although 'I' can learn to skate board, or 'I' may be on acid - 'I' am still 'I'. It is difficult, and may well be philosophically impossible, to say what this sense of 'I' is. Where does this 'narrative centre of gravity' come from? Within the functional polarity of autism/schizophrenia the 'I' might be thought of as the autistic tendency within each of us. We see ourselves as unitary beings, acted on by events in a pretty much logical, sequential manner. Whereas when we become different we make a previously 'Other' aspect of the world (e.g. the pointer on the computer monitor) relate directly to our sense of 'I'.

There are thousands of psychological and cognitive experiments that show the tendency that we have to confabulate in order to support our sense of 'I' continuity. A classic example is the phenomena of 'negative hallucination'.[139] If a person is hypnotised and told that there is no furniture in the room, when asked to fetch something from the far corner of the room they will still avoid the furniture. If asked why they did not walk straight to the corner subjects respond with false statements (e.g. 'I noticed a picture on the wall and moved to look at it'). The strange thing is that, even thought we know that our sense of 'I' is full of confabulation and gaps, I still have a pretty good chance of remembering what I look like in a mirror (even though I am different in some small way, every day) and where I left my house keys.

We are left with a fundamental paradox - namely that the Self is both schizophrenic and autistic - both tending towards seeing the Other as potentially part of itself, and at the same time seeking a continuity of experience as separate. 'I' am fluid and can change. 'I' can become different, through learning, and extending and altering the boundaries between Self and Other. Equally 'I' seek to exist as a unitary being, as me, and to organise my various experiences into a linear narrative that is 'my history'.

## Dawn of the Iconoclast

Transgression, in one sense, is the process through which we generate new experiences, it is the process of slipping between Self and Other and redefining the boundaries of knowledge and understanding.

Unlike a computer, our universe is not bounded by rules that are written from outside. Rather our rules are human constructions from within the 'game' of reality. This does not only include codified laws that prohibit incest or require us not to double park, it also includes a social context that defines how we think of our ourselves (male, middle-class, sane, bisexual etc.) and assumptions that determine how much control we believe we have over the world (I believe that I can only see with my eyes, that my arm is under my control, while the balloon in the sky is not).

Transgression means the breaking of these 'laws', and drug experience, especially drug experience that tends toward the numinous or self-actualising, is a powerful method of transgression.

In one sense, transgression may imply law-breaking in the conventional sense of the term. It can imply the sort of iconoclastic, taboo breaking activities used by devotees of the Vama Marg (or 'Left Hand Path') Tantrik cults.[140] Within Hindu society taboo breaking might mean drinking wine out of a human skull, eating beef, swallowing semen etc.[141] Certainly within society today there are too many taboos that can be a powerful, self-transformative experience to break. Indeed the very act of using drugs (whether for recreational or magical purposes) is itself taboo. However the law-breaking aspect of transgression has often been overstated, especially by the outré followers of post-modern philosophy and art.

Any taboo breaking aspect of transgression must seek not only to establish what is taboo but why the taboo is broken and for whom. The transgressor should be aware that in order to rebel one needs not only something to rebel against but something to rebel towards. The psychoanalysist Lacan describes this as the 'ideal ego' (what you seek to be by undertaking a certain course of action) and the 'ego ideal' (the place from which you imagine that your actions are being watched). So, to transgress in order to become a fuller and more authentic Self might be a good thing, but if the ego ideal of the transgression is, say your reproachful father, then the transgression itself is fatally flawed. In short the transgressor must ask not simply 'what will I become if I break such-and-such a taboo', but also 'why or for what ego ideal (for whom) am I breaking it?'

There is another equally important feature of transgression that must be understood. Transgression would simply be the cult of the 'bigger and better buzz' unless it were for the fact that taboo breaking need not literally mean doing that which is not, literally, lawful. Transgression means to deliberately enter into the realm of the schizophrenic, the world where impressions and experiences fall on the Self and either obliterate the sense of 'I' (as with the numinous experience), or serve to provide impressions of the world that are not mediated by the usual laws of language and meaning. For instance the experience of seeing a sunset, really seeing it and participating in it, being caught up in it rather than passively observing it - this can be as much an act of transgression as anything else.

## Back to Life, Back to Reality

The shamanic return is vital. It is the precarious path from the schizophrenia realm of the Other, back into the autistic realm of the sequential universe. Even within the deepest datura trance, the blindness of the belladonna, and the peak of the peyote vision, it is possible to make out and take the path of the shamanic return. The return from the new state of consciousness that transgression itself permits is itself an act of transgression. Since the Self has been obliterated into the schizophrenic void of chaos, the act of re-capturing the autistic, linear narrative of the self itself transgresses madness and gives that which is beyond meaning, meaning.

For the philosopher Hegel this process, what he identified as the 'production of objective knowledge' through the dialectic, was the basic process of discovering truth. For individuals like George Bataille and Nietzsche, the aim was rather a submerging of Self in the anti-gnosis of the subjective. Personally I see both processes (the schizophrenic merging with the Other and the shamanic return to the autistic fiction of the objective Self) as an inseparable part of the whole.

The shaman[142] talks with the spirits of the dead, he is stripped of his skin by carrion crows, he must fuck his mother to receive magical powers and then he must return. He is certainly changed but still he has *returned*.

The distinction between the shaman and magician (or between the transcendental and the immanent) is, as mentioned above, a false one. Whether we transgress through ritual spells, drugs or arduous programs of meditation, we must reach outward towards the Other and then return again to the centre of the Self (to begin once more...).

One must be able to transgress 'into' the sunset and relate to it in a way that subverts or is outside of normal human language and laws. Yet the magician (which I think is the best term for someone who can perform such feats of transgression with style and skill) must also be able to say 'ah, look at that wonderful sunset' and make it an objective part of her universe.

In philosophical terms drug experience is a transgression that reveals the 'real' existence outside of the symbolic realm (that we inhabit in day-to-day being and culture). This timeless, numinous moment is Maslow's 'peak experience'. Although we speak of it as a 'moment' it is literally *outside of time*. Equally we talk of making a 'shamanic return' from the real, yet we are never really apart from it. In the language of Hermetic occultism the real is the 'circle whose centre is everywhere and whose circumference is nowhere found'. In terms of our functional polarity, of autism and schizophrenia, numinous experience plays across the meaninglessness of autistic being and the hypermeaningfulness of schizophrenia.

## One of Us Must Know

The flux and flow of ourselves (our functional polarity of schizophrenia and autistism) and processes (transgression/reintegration) provides some useful insight into a fundamental problem of western philosophy. To put the problem simply: we live in a world of shared experience and meaning. The very existence of language and culture demonstrate as much. Yet at the same time, if we examine our descriptions of the world (as post-modern philosophy does) we often find that what we thought was common turns out to be widely divergent. My experience of any text (and remember a text can be thought of practically any form of experience, not just writing) will be different given my culture, race, gender, sexual orientation, period of history, etc.[143]

The drive towards relativism, even a nihilistic relativism as exemplified by British broadsheet journalism in the late 1980s, can seem like the logical outcome of post-modernism. After all perhaps if our relationships and readings of texts (our discourses) can be so different, can we really be said to live in a homogenous world?

Philosophical schools such as phenomenology attempted to answer this problem by suggesting that we occupy a 'real' world but that we see it from many different perspectives. Phenomenology attempts to try to discover this 'real world' by analysing texts and trying to draw out the fundamental features, those experiences that were 'primary' and not mediated by preconceptions. In this way primary experiences could be identified by 'bracketing out'[144] prejudices so that the pure phenomenon (the object of experience *in itself*) could be known.

There are a number of objections to both the phenomenological and relativist-post-modernist approaches. However I see the model of Self that I have proposed as being able to accommodate both observations (namely, that there is a real world but it can appear radically differently for different people). Part of the resolution is that that there does not have to be only one answer. As Derrida and other philosophers have pointed out, there is a marked tendency for western philosophy to look for the solution. Just as our physicists are looking for the grand unified theory of everything, so our culture tends to want a unitary, simple and concrete solution. Yet as our examination of drug experience shows, the same drug can have simultaneously remarkably similar and also radically different effects.

Perhaps human experience is closer to the model of the 'holon' proposed by Arthur Koestler[145] rather than the monolithic one truth our culture tries to demand. A holon is a system that exhibits the simultaneous tendencies to remain whole in itself, and to seek to be a part of something greater. Thus a human cells seeks to maintain its integrity as an individual cell, but also seeks to be part of a whole body.

Drug experience demonstrates how humans are holons. We have a shared experience of drug states[146] and yet our experiences can be widely divergent. We can experience the world so that we place all meaning in 'the Other' (the schizophrenic mode of perception), and we can place all meaning within ourselves only (the autistic model). What is important to us as humans is maintaining our fluidity between these modes of being. It is this flow of meaning, through the processes of transgression and reintegration that allows us to have both shared values and cultural difference; a common lived-in world and perspectival diversity.

## (Refining your) Rapture

Let's begin to focus on the actual use of drugs in an occult context, and look at specific practices and processes. In order to appreciate these stories of drug experience in action there are a few points that need to be understood at the outset. Especially for those who have not used, or who are new to the notion of using drugs as a form of magical transgression.

One important point that I'll mention straight off is simply this: 'more isn't necessarily better'. There is a macho view that somehow taking 500 micrograms of LSD makes you cooler, more 'out there', wiser or simply 'harder' than somebody who gets loaded on 100 micrograms.[147] Apart from the mere fact that different people react to drugs in different ways (and that their reactions can differ because of a wide range of factors), a larger dose does not necessarily mean a greater act of transgression or a more profound experience. Each individual finds his or her own optimum dose of a given drug. For some people this may mean nothing, since the drug simply doesn't agree with them physiologically or psychologically. For some the dose may be relatively high, for others an appreciation of the drug effect may be developed so as to 'refine your rapture'. What I mean by this is that, by altering variables such as dosage, set and setting and tolerance to a given drug, a greater effect can be had with less chemical. Now this is not to say that there is some puritan benefit in being able to enter the numinous with less chemical assistance. Rather the idea is that when you take drugs, especially for transformative purposes, the experience should be a powerful one. It is a question of preparing optimum conditions for such a powerful experience to manifest.

Let me give you an example from my own experience. I enjoy smoking skunk. I enjoy the smell, the gentle mushroom like sense of trippy disassociation that skunk gives me. I also find that I develop a tolerance to skunk quite quickly. This means that if I want a powerful skunk effect I have to either switch strains (from smoking say 'northern lights' to using 'purple haze') or I have to reduce my consumption so that I become re-sensitised to the drug, or I have to change my set and setting in such a way to make full use of the skunk hit (perhaps by smoking within a ritual or party context). So, I know from my own experience that if I want to make good use of skunk as a drug I need to 'refine my rapture'. In other words rather than simply taking more and more of the drug I realise which effects I like and seek to enhance these by reducing my consumption and altering the environment within which I take the drug.

If nothing else the attitude of simply taking more and more, smacks of capitalist consumer culture rather than an intelligent approach to drug use. Moreover the effect of most drugs changes in relation to tolerance. For instance many psychoactives simply will not work (or will have very little effect) if they are taken too often. Even increasing the dosage will not overcome this. Other drugs are such that a large dose may result in effects which come from the chemical being at near toxic levels within the body, or may cause additional effects that are unwanted (for instance large doses of datura[148] can cause temporary blindness, while drugs like nutmeg, taken in large doses, may cause kidney damage).

Having a transformative interaction with drugs may mean experimenting with a number of chemicals, or it may mean developing a close and respectful relationship with just one or two. It may mean experiments in high doses but one should never confuse the simple quantity of the dose with the power of the experience. Factors like set and setting, the placebo effect and one's own sensitivity to the drug experience must always be born in mind. These variables are just as, if not more important than, quantity.

If 'I' am to have a powerful and meaningful drug experience I have got to take enough to allow my sense of 'I' to be destroyed (or at least significantly altered). However, in order to make the shamanic return 'I' must allow my sense of Self to return and not loose sight of it. Put simply, if you take so much that you don't remember anything about it, are you really having an enjoyable or interesting time? Certainly there may be aspects or types of drug experience that are wholly 'Other' in the sense that they cannot be easily brought back into waking consciousness. Now these experiences still inform who we are, in the same way that dreams that we don't remember in the morning are still part of our memory, our being, our 'I'. 'Losing it' can certainly be valuable, but it can often be a flight away from experience rather than an intelligent attempt to broaden it. The reason that drugs get used to excess (in this sense) is usually because the drug taker's life is so grim that they are simply seeking escape. This is a faster or slower (depending on which drug one chooses) road to suicide. Escape from the world through drugs may be a legitimate project, but it is rarely an empowering one.

Although a detailed discussion of addiction is outside the scope of this book the relationship between drugs and addiction is an important one. Although the term addiction is increasingly used in more general contexts (such as 'sex addiction' or 'shopping addiction'), it is generally 'substance addiction' that is meant, usually where the substance concerned is a drug.

A better way of looking at addiction is to look at it as an addiction to an *experience*. In the case of drugs this means the whole ritual surrounding the obtaining, use, effects and broader context within which the experience is framed. Most drug agencies with a policy of 'harm reduction' (rather than 'just say no') are keenly aware that drug addiction is by no means only about using a substance.

Psychoanalysts too, who have worked with drug addicts, recognise that drug use need not necessarily imply abuse, even when the drug is one that can be very seductive;

> The term 'drug initiate' would thus refer to that hypothetical individual who doesn't *abuse* drugs, but who *uses* them as a mean of satisfying his innate, archetypal need for initiation...'drug initiate' is a concept, a hypothetical ideal impossible to achieve in the context of our consumerist culture.[149]

In contrast to the psychoanalyst Zoja's comment above, I feel that it is possible to be a drug initiate (though it is an ongoing process of initiation, and not a final state). But he is right to suggest that one must escape from consumerist culture (to some degree) in order to use drugs intelligently.

Since drugs experiences are liminal, both 'outside' (setting) and 'inside' (set), they can become the gateways to healing (through medical use, therapy or self-actualisation). As things from 'outside' the self, drugs can provide much needed support. Prozac, for instance, is an excellent drug for some people to give them a breathing space, outside of depression, where they can begin again to take control of their lives. Drugs can be life rafts that help those in trauma. This can range from the medical prescription of antidepressants to the self medication of getting drunk to 'forget' and pass through the pain of an ended relationship. But 'going on a bender', or overusing one drug to extricate oneself not from a specific situation, but from one's whole life means that addiction is just around the corner. Drug addiction is like obsessively keeping a key that you know is important, but having forgotten the door that it unlocks. With drugs the danger is that one's whole being, body and mind, becomes familiar with the substance(s) and so the drug loses its effect and is reduced to simply maintaining 'normal' psychological and physiological function. In this case the key has found the lock and imprisoned the drug user.

# Blood, Sugar, Sex, Magick: drugs in esoteric culture

## Superstructure

We have already met the Indian Tantrik tradition in terms of taboo breaking transgression. Tantra represents the Indian equivalent of much of the European esoteric traditions, and much of the occult tantrik teaching that deals with the sacred use of drugs. These teachings include the use of a range of substances, many of which few modern people would readily classify as drugs. These include materials which might properly be thought of as acting in a homeopathic or purely occult manner (such as the ashes of burnt cow dung, water drawn from holy places and so on). Most notably of all Tantrik 'drugs' include the use of human secretions. This area, which is collectively known as the study of the 'kalas' (which may be variously translated as 'times', 'colours' or 'poisons and nectars') has been the subject of only a few relatively obscure western occult authors.[150]

The kalas are 'subtle chemicals' that may be present in a number of different human secretions - urine, shit, semen, menstrual fluid and love juice. According to the tantrik teachings these substances - depending on how they are generated and collected - may be imbued with fantastic powers.

There is a vigorous (though actively suppressed) tradition of using sexual and other secretions for magical purposes (often as aphrodisiacs) in the west. For instance Bourchard, Bishop of Worms in an Episcopal letter writes that;

> ..some women are want to do...they take their menstrual blood and mix it with food or drink, and give it to their men to consume or imbibe, in order to expect more from them...They prostrate themselves on their faces, and with their buttocks open they order bread to be prepared over their naked arses, and when this has been mixed they con their husbands into eating it.[151].

According to western science many of these substances do indeed contain important amino-acids and endocrine secretions. There is evidence, for instance, that drinking one's own urine can serve to set up a feedback loop within the body which makes the drinker more sensitive to certain 'dark senses'.[152] We also have indigenous traditions with an advanced knowledge of using odour to produce drug effects; amongst these are the 'Horse Whisperers'. The Horse Whisperers were a semi-secret organisation, active throughout the British Isles. An initiated tradition of men who used a knowledge of herbs and secretions to magically control horses.

The more esoteric uses of the kalas in Tantra remind us that it isn't only the substance as much as the set, the setting and the way that it is generated that is important. For instance, a tantrik priestess might secrete the kalas within her vaginal fluid, but certain kalas will only be produced if she is being sexually stimulated in a certain way, and at a particular time within her menstrual cycle. Moreover to have its desired effect, the vaginal mucus may need to be consumed in a particular way (in some traditions licked off a bay leaf, in others swallowed on a wafer, in others drink directly from the cunt of the priestess). The alleged effects of the kalas are manifold, ranging from increased sensory abilities to far more dramatic occult skills (such as providing one with precognitive insight or rendering one immune to all poisons).

Obviously the idea that magical or transformative power can be contained within sexual fluids has given rise to some serious misunderstandings of Tantrism. As with any drug we should concentrate on the experience and not simply the commodity. To think of the kalas as the esoteric equivalent of monkey gland treatment for old age is like confusing the wine of the mass with the alcohol you might use to disinfect a cut.[153] Although the material might be the same, the context, the meaning and the experience of the two drugs is quite different.

Since the kalas are substances that straddle the boundary between drug/not drug, sacred/profane and organic/inorganic they certainly exist, in a cultural sense, as liminal materials. What we do currently know is that some drugs (notably psychoactives) do remain active in body fluids produced by the drug taker. The classic example of this is the Siberian shamanic practice of drinking urine from people who have eaten psychedelic mushrooms. From a strict biological point of view the same practice should be possible with a number of other psychoactive compounds. It would certainly be interesting to know if these drugs are secreted in other body fluids, notably the sexual ones. It may be that a synergy takes place between the internal state of the person (producing hormones) and a drug secreted in their sex fluids. What such endocrine substances (psychedelic kalas) would do it remains for magicians to explore.

## Whatever Gets you Through the Night

The Story of the kalas demonstrates another aspect of the liminality of drugs. Since it is not simply semen that the Tantrik worshipper swallows, but rather sacred semen produced by the incarnation of the god Shiva, ejaculated as the result of specific erotic ritual, and drunk in a sacred manner. These Tantrik 'drugs' are not only substances, indeed most of what makes them sacred is the situation, the set and setting, surrounding them.

This reiterates my point that the definition of drug experience is actually so blurred that it can include virtually anything.[154] After all, if drinking sacred menstrual blood can change my hormonal system, if taking a pill of placebo morphine can reduce my pain, and if my experience of acid can be profoundly altered by my set and setting - where and what is the actual power of the drug?

Across time and culture people have used many methods of sacred transgression. These include techniques which undoubtedly alter one's own neurochemistry and, in the broadest sense, engender 'drug experience'. Various commentators on shamanism argue for the primacy of either psychedelic or ordeal based shamanism. Personally I believe that the distinction itself is somewhat false. Some commentators have suggested that 'ordeal based' shamanism (where numinous experiences are sought through drumming, fasting, ritual drama, pain etc.) are later developments designed to compensate for the fact that humans migrated out of areas in which psychedelic plants grew in great abundance.[155] Personally I find this doubtful, especially since we have examples of extreme ordeal based methods (such as the feats of physical edurance witnessed at the sundance ceremony) which exist in parallel to the use of psychedelics (i.e. peyote) within the same native American cultures.[156] Also there is no reason ancient humans could not have used other plants (there are very few, if any, areas of the world where psychedelic and other powerful drugs are not available) or, if they were really so important, have maintained trade links for these substances or indeed learnt to cultivate them.[157]

Many techniques of changing consciousness can be combined together in different ways and for different purposes. Formal ritual or psychodrama, in my experience, works well only with moderate doses of drugs (i.e. hashish and alcohol). Whereas for psychedelics breath control and drumming blend really well. Techniques involving pain and eroticism can benefit from small amounts of the gentler drugs, although it may be that, as new drugs are developed and discovered, new possibilities and permutations emerge.

One example of this is 2-CB, a drug from the same chemical family as MDMA. 2-CB appears to act on the limbic system, the 'reptilian' hind brain, in small doses it acts as a somatic hallucinogen (enhancing smell and touch) and may be useful for erotic experiments. In higher doses it appears to stimulate the 'fight, fright, flight' responses, leading to a sense of an all encompassing 'animal fear'[158] which might be of interest to those magicians experimenting with pain or terror as a method of transgression[159].

## Walking on the Edge

As well as numinous experience being possible from ordeal or ritualised practices it can also occur apparently unbidden and without warning. Although we might retrospectively discern the patterns in an individual's life that lead to 'spontaneous' mystical experience, this analysis is generally well after the fact.

In tribal cultures it is often illness that precipitates the shamanic journey and the experience of being near death, whether through disease or injury, certainly carries with it transformative potential. However for other people these experiences simply come 'unbidden'. A common category of spontaneous numinous experience is the 'childhood nature mystery experience'.[160] This type of experience is recounted by writer Kenneth Rexroth, magician Giordano Bruno (1548-1600) and famously by C.S.Lewis:

> As I stood beside a flowering currant bush on a summer day there suddenly arose in me without warning…a sensation…[it] is difficult to find words strong enough for the sensation which came over me; Milton's 'enormous bliss' of Eden…comes somewhere near it…It had taken only a moment of time; and in a certain sense everything else that had ever happened to me was insignificant in comparison.

Since the intentionality of the 'I' is subverted during a spontaneous mystical experience we should perhaps not be altogether surprised that many such experiences are terrifying rather than beatific. As an example of this, one very different form of transgressive event that occurs in modern culture, is a constellation of experiences that have become know as 'alien abduction'.

The phenomena of alien abduction is fascinating. In essence I believe that it represents, in at least some cases, a genuine visitation of individuals by beings from another reality. This does not mean physical space aliens are abducting people.[161] Rather I believe that these beings may be expressions of forces that exist within our unconscious minds.[162] They may be archetypal images, in the mould of Jung who proposed that UFOs were the current cultural expression of spirit entities, angels and gods. Drawing distinctions as to whether they are 'images that express unconscious content' or 'real' denizens of an unseen realm (which most shamanic belief systems postulate) is pretty meaningless. The point is that these beings are experienced as though they were independent of our normal consciousness, yet they seem to undoubtedly come clothed in the prejudices and symbolism of the culture in which they manifest. This last feature is so true that today, in the last years of the 20th century, we even have a standardised image of the alien (viz. 'the grey' of *Close Encounters* and the *X-Files*).

Many, though by no means all, alien abductions have a frightening content. Often they include forced surgery or 'tests', sometimes with distinctly sexual overtones. Interesting, on the other end of the equation, we have the celebrated 'alien autopsy' footage of an alleged alien cadaver recovered in the USA.[163] Thus not only do the aliens examine us, but we too dissect them.

Read symbolically the dissection motif might be telling our culture a lot about our attitude to the 'Other' or innerworld. We are obsessed with dissecting it (using reductive, autistic methods such as materialist science). We are worried that 'the alien' may carry us away, outside not only of space but also of time. We often fear them, sometimes we seek salvation from them, either way become lost in a mass of conspiracy theory since we insist on having some way to make rational sense of their actions.

The type of experiences reported by abductees closely parallels experience reported by many users of the powerful tryptamine hallucinogen DMT. Moreover encounters that, allowing for cultural difference, sound remarkably parallel to abductions can be found amongst tribal people who use the tryptamine based ayahuasca preparation. Reports of apparently external, intelligent 'alien' or sometimes 'fairy' beings are common with DMT hallucinations.[164]

Briefly stated, I believe that some cases of alien abduction might be the result of spontaneous DMT experiences. DMT occurs endogenously and it may well be that certain environmental or psychological effects might raise levels in the body (or the mind's sensitivity) so that a DMT-type trip results.[165]

Electro-magnetic or other 'dark sensory' events (set and setting) may be sufficient to create an endogenous DMT trip. There is some evidence, from the research of Dr Susan Blackmore, that electro-magnetism can create hallucinatory states, some of which sound fairly close to abduction experiences.[166]

Leaving aside the details of the DMT and aliens enquiry, it is certainly the case that environmental factors, the effects on our bodies and brains that our 'dark senses' register, can provoke states akin to drug experiences. In this way we can begin to think of a broader approach to the setting of drug experience. Our bodies are continually enmeshed in a web of charged particles, scent, pressure, tiny gravitational and electromagnetic changes. Perhaps there are other, more subtle and pervasive forces, which western science does not have the necessarily instrumentation to measure but that we are unconsciously aware of. This being the case, perhaps circumstances can conspire to bring on a drug-like experience where no actual drug has been taken. Perhaps also this model could explain why two separate people might have similar visions (say, in the case of a UFO close encounter). Since it is not only a brain event, but one provoked by a common set of environmental conditions. The sense of sharing an experience, or possessing a drug induced telepathy, may operate in just the same way for endogenously produced trips.

## Medicine Bow

The liminal realm, which drugs are both of, and may allow access to, is central in esoteric symbolism. As we have already seen, the figure of the witch or shaman occupies this realm. The gender of the shaman may be ambiguous, the witch may symbolically live on the boundary between the civilisation of the village and the unknown darkness of the wild wood.

The liminal makes repeated appearances in magic. For example, traditionally magical rituals are conducted within a circle. The circle itself may be drawn upon the earth or simply made, by an act of 'organised imagination',[167] perhaps by drawing a blade through the air. Whatever way it is formed, the magic circle has three main functions. Firstly, it prevents hostile spirits from disrupting the magician's work. Secondly, it forms a sealed area within which magical energy (of the type desired) can be built up, in somewhat the same manner as charging an electrical battery. Thirdly, the circle exists, as Wiccan ritual expresses it 'in this place that is not a place, in this time that is not a time, between the realm of humans and of the gods'. In other words the circle is a liminal place; it partakes of both worlds but exists ('plays') between them. The magician can therefore explore and affect both worlds, by having a foot in both camps but remaining bound by the rules of neither sphere.

In the same way a ritual may be designed to take place at an 'in-betweenness' time. Midnight is the classic witching hour, in that it is between one day and the next. Some witches I know use dawn or dusk for just the same reason; that the world is shifting from darkness to light (or vice versa). Other times of transgressive power include the sabbats, or pagan festivals. These include the solstices and equinoxes and the folk festivals of Imbolc, Beltain, Lammas and Samhain.[168] The most well-loved of these dates tend to be May Eve (Beltain) and Halloween

(Samhain). In both cases occult lore claims that the 'veil between the worlds becomes thinner'. On May Eve the burgeoning forces of sexuality are beginning to flood outward from the underworld of winter (hence the blossoming of the Hawthorne or May). At Halloween the inhabitance of the overworld turn their faces again towards the coming darkness and winter, and the spirits of the ancestors are abroad.

Rituals that seek to transgress the world and enter the liminal state may include acts of initiation, of passing through symbolic doors[169] or of invoking the help of spirits who are 'guardians of the portals'.[170] The symbolism of the shaman 'making the crossing' or 'walking between the worlds'[171] is exceedingly complex, rich and pervasive. (Whether we are considering the offerings left for Hecate, the Goddess of the Witches, at the crossroads, the reversal of symbolic or social roles within traditional Wicca,[172] or the use of the 'special attitude' by contemporary magicians i.e. that 'the gods' are both real *and* imaginary at the same time).[173] In all these cases the aim is to consciously enter the liminal sphere, to 'go between', and thereby be free to alter one's awareness, to learn new perspectives, to understand better, and perhaps change both inner and outer universes.

In order to facilitate drug experience, the intelligent user will explore methods of entering the liminal sphere that are synergistic with the particular drug, and desired experience. The study and use of these techniques is the art and science of magic.

## Me and My Charms

By changing our consciousness we can access all manner of abilities, skills, insights and understanding which I refer to as 'magical powers'. Magic is generally perceived as being deeply anti-rational, supernatural and unknowable. Yet magic also implies the use of ritual, symbolic languages, ceremony, and perhaps complex metaphysics. In fact magic contains both the deeply irrational and the complex formulaic at once and therefore maintains the same liminal duality or paradox as drug experience.

Although we might consider drugs using scientific language (when we talk about synapses, neuropharmacology and so on), in the western world it is the irrational world of the schizophrenic that we are most estranged from. And so it is the unconscious, the right-hemisphere, the serotonin 'Other' reality, that drugs are most often used to gain access to. We live our lives in a way that exults the sequential and the orderly, and fears the irrational and the chaotic.

The following is an examination of particular drugs along with my personal experiences and insights drawn from talking to others that have experimented with these drugs. Some of the experiences that I have had and heard of are, without doubt, shamanic or magical. Although I will show how some scientific findings may be linked with certain occult phenomena, I do not propose that they can easily be explained in scientific terms. If you wish to disregard these experiences as fanciful or wishful thinking then that is fine, if you wish to think of them as 'symbolic' but not 'real', then that's fine too.[174] I tend to think of these things as magical, that is they are not above suspicion or analysis (indeed the essence of the shamanic return is the ability to make sense of these experiences). However there may simply be some things that resist analysis into general principles or 'laws'. In the same way we do not know what 'laws' determine the content of dreams, yet from ancient times, until Freud and after, the content of dreams has been seen as being useful in analysing the past, present and future of the dreamer. We do not know how dreaming works, but that need not stop us from being open to the suggestion that dreaming is useful and perhaps carries meaning on a whole variety of different levels.

Finally for those people who would dismiss the occult power of drugs as intoxicated delusion I have one point to add.

It is quite possible, though by no means certain, that since the dawn of humanity we have used drugs to explore the invisible realms. These forays have gained humanity a wealth of knowledge. For some tribes the use of drugs has absolutely pragmatic reasons. The intoxicated shaman may be able to heal the sick, travel over vast distances in search of game, to steal the souls of enemies, to commune with vegetation spirits in order to know which plants in a new region are good to eat. If theorists such as Wasson and McKenna are right, much of the very basis of the human psyche and even language may be traced to interactions between humans and drugs. If these things were all fantasy would they have such a venerable, widespread and still-utilised currency? Moreover would not humanity have simply sidled off into an evolutionary blind alley, made mad and unfit to survive because of our naive misconception that plants could literally teach us? Perhaps, as more than one ethnographer has noted, the fault may be in us, and not due to the imagined foolishness of tribal peoples. The Sanema Indians told the anthropologist Johannes Wilbert that their shamans could fly, or at least walk one foot above the ground. Naively, the scientist answered that after all, he could *see* that the shamans ran around just like anybody else. Whereupon the Indians countered, 'The reason for that is that you do not *understand.*'

I suspect that materialist science is far from the whole truth (though I would not wish to reject it as one amongst a host of invaluable tools for investigating the world). The history of shamanic practice, and most importantly personal experience, leads to me to believe that not only is drug experience legitimate as a way of mystical illumination, it is also a gateway to magical powers.

Let us now examine these powers in more detail.

## Preparing to Fly

For witches and shamans magical flight goes with the territory. Indeed the experience of 'getting high' (in a literal sense) is, I believe, much more common than many people suppose. A number of drugs seem to be closely associated with flight, these include datura, ayahuasca, and henbane. The psychedelic disassociative ketamine also commonly provokes flying dreams.

Flying tends to be an important part of shamanic, tribal traditions and may include flying over 'real' landscape, as well as flying through other worlds (such as flying under the ground, or under the ocean and meeting symbolic creatures).[175] In practice, the distinction seems to be of little real importance since the world of spirits and the world of humans mutually interpenetrate each other. For the shaman in her trance it may be possible to observe both 'actual' events happening some distance away as well as to observe the movements of spirit creatures and other denizens of the invisible realm.

In many cultures there is a blurred distinction too between whether the shaman 'actually' flies, or flies 'in spirit'. In some cultures the shaman will retire alone into a hut before leaving his body and flying. In other situations[176] the flight takes place before witnesses and, though the physical body of the witch remains motionless on the floor, never the less she has flown.

For the shaman the proof of the flight rests less in whether his body flies, than in whether what he sees in the flying vision is accurate and useful. As neuropathology records, it is certainly possible for the sense of 'I' to become located outside of the physical body (or located within an 'astral' or imaginary body which is not limited by the location of the physical body). This ability to locate the self outside of the physical form is, I believe, a vital procedure in shamanic flight. However it does nothing to explain how, from a materialist perspective, the mind can be projected across space in order to observe actual incidents taking place at a distance. This phenomena, whether it is called 'astral projection' or 'remote viewing' is a fundamental part of esoteric lore and I believe is an ability that is accessible given the correct conditions (with or without drugs).

Over the years I have spoken to a number of people who have experienced shamanic flight as part of a drug experience. The most common experience is of a genuine corporeal sense of flying. This is usually over familiar landscape but from an unfamiliar vantage point, that is usually no more than a few hundred feet up in the air. For most people it seems that the whole event is 'realistic', although for some people, flying through time as well as space and experiencing the mythic world (i.e. a landscape populated with spirits and strange entities) overlaid on the 'actual world' is not unknown. Most people that I've spoken to have only had a single flying vision. To date I have only had one spontaneous LSD associated flying vision. This is despite the fact that I have used astral projection techniques, 'borrowing'[177] and lucid dreaming methods (with some reasonable success).

The ability to travel 'in spirit vision' relies heavily on the imagination. Indeed many occultists of the modern period argue that in order to develop such a radical ability the critical faculties of the mind must be temporarily silenced. The occultists W B Leadbeater, Aleister Crowley and others suggest that, at least in the initial stages of many occult practices, the critical faculties (the autistic mode of consciousness) do more harm than good.[178] The process of suspending judgement is necessary to deal with the fact that, according to 'common sense', people simply do not fly. So whether it is possible that we can make forays with our sense of awareness outside of our bodies, our cultural conditioning is that this simply cannot be true. Therefore the magician begins in a spirit of playfulness, of 'what if...', of uncritical fancy.[179] This is not to say that this attitude remains throughout one's experiments with magical flight, or indeed is pervasive throughout occultism. In fact during the 19th century organisations such as the Hermetic Order of the Golden Dawn[180] developed a series of methods for supposedly determining just how 'pure' or accurate a spirit vision was (by close analysis of symbols and colours in the 'vision' that were compared with the system of correspondences used in *Qabalah*). Moreover, the magician, once the technique is learnt, is encouraged to discover various ways of testing and examining the process itself.[181]

This way of learning is quite the antithesis of the scientific method. Rather than using a deductive dialectic, which starts with a hypothesis about the world, and then seeks to test it through experiments, the magical way is almost the reverse. A possibility is played with 'as if' it were true. Then in time it may become true. Finally, the relative merit or truth of the experience is subjected to analysis from as many different directions as possible.

Perhaps, like the results of remote viewing experiments conducted by the US Military during the cold war, we may find convincing evidence that the mind (that elusive fiction) can be projected through time, space and layers of reality. As John Wyndham points out in his novel *Chocky* 'mind has no mass', and this being so, perhaps the limitations that physics places on space travel may really be a figment of our imaginations.

Duerr explains that shamanic 'flying' is not the same as the process of moving through the air as we usually conceive of it;

> ...as *brujo* [sorcerer] need not be able to fly like a bird in order to arrive at a different place within seconds, for it seems that a sorcerer can change boundaries of his person so much that he can be simultaneously within his everyday body and *also* at another place, where his body is not. Something like this may indeed be happening during divination and telepathy...It does not seem to be a transmission as assumed by most parapsychologists. We are apparently dealing more with a 'lifting of boundaries', in which there is a dissolution of barriers developed during the process of civilization and individuation.

He goes on to record the account of one ethnographer's drug experiment, which led to a successful flying vision;

> The body that I had left behind lay in the boat as if dead. I myself, my astral body or whatever you want to call it started floating. A thought or a wish was sufficient to take me wherever I wanted to go. All movement was accompanied by euphoric feelings of pleasure. I wished myself to the nearest tree – and there I was. When I grabbed the trunk of the tree, it remained in my hand, or rather, it went through my hand. Then I floated through the tree trunk, or perhaps I should say; the tree went through me while I moved forward. I now realised that I could wish myself to whatever place I pleased, and so I wished myself to the nearest Walpurgis-Night orgy. Instantly I was there.

> The picture that presented itself to me was indescribable. Naked women of unspeakable beauty floated about. Were they fairies, goddesses, demonesses? I don't know.

> I joined the dance, wished myself to the naked fairy that seemed

the most gorgeous to me. Her sensuous charm surpassed description – and I united with her...[182]

The flight of the shaman brings with it the knowledge of new perspectives, both literally and figuratively. The flight is in the inner world and perhaps the outerworld also. As the boundaries between Self and Other are dissolved in the drug experience it becomes possible to travel without moving.

## Transformer

The power of shamanic flight is often coupled with the ability to borrow the form of, or indeed to fully become, a flying creature. We have, for example, the classic account of a woman turning into a bird from *The Golden Ass* by Lucius Apuleius;

> ...a small cabinet containing several little boxes, one of which she opened. It contained an ointment which she worked about with her fingers and then smeared all over her body from the soles of her feet to the crown of her head. After this she muttered a long charm to her lamp, and shook herself; and, as I watched her limbs become gradually fledged with feather, her arms changed into sturdy wings, her nose grew crooked, and horny, her nails turned into talons, and soon there was no longer any doubt about it: Pamphilë had become an owl. She gave a querulous hoot and made a few little hopping flights until she was sure enough of her wings to glide off, away over the roof-tops.

As Peter Duerr points out in *Dreamtime*,[183] it does not make sense to ask if the witch really becomes a bird. The answer will depend in what sense you are prepared to adjudge the transformation as real.

In the language of science some 98% of human DNA is identical to that of the great apes, while of this figure some 40-odd percent is identical with that of a tree. In more expressive language, the world of animals is the world of our relations. We are different from them, but not necessarily any better (again the question rests on from where one wishes to measure our assumed superiority). Although we as human creatures may feel more empathy with a dog than with a sea slug, that is really no reason to imagine that the inner life of the sea slug is less complex or valuable. Many of the criteria that we usually measure our superiority by may be little more than functional specialisations. Humans create technologies, whilst whales sing songs and beavers build dams - which is better?

The magical formula[184] known as Atavistic Resurgence is a modern re-statement of the power of transformation of form that is an integral part of shaman stories and witch lore. Atavistic resurgence suggests that humans can tap the powers of the other creatures that share our planet. Once again, as with shamanic flight, this might be imagined as a shifting of the location of 'I' from the human realm to something Other; something animal.

Atavistic resurgence was described by Austin Osman Spare, one of the foremost western occultists of the 20th century.[185] Spare used a system of sexual magic, breath control and artistic techniques to summon 'atavisms' from within.[186] These latent animal powers (which might be the 'real' power of the creature - e.g. the strength of the tiger, or an 'imagined' power - e.g. the wisdom of the owl) could be summoned by Spare's highly personal system of sorcery. In this way Spare stands firmly within the shamanic complex of practices.

The transgression of the human/other boundary in drug experience can allow us to communicate with animals, it can allow us to experience them as teachers. Spirit animals may attend the shaman in her journeys into the innerworld. These creatures may be allies, providing counsel or special abilities which may assist the shaman's quest. Alternatively the witch may become the hare, seeking out information with her highly trained senses, hiding and observing, perhaps sneaking under the hedge of culture to plant curses or blessings as she desires.

If one has never had the experience of identification with, or of becoming another creature, simple interactions with another animal within the drug experience can be profoundly rewarding. I recall one wet afternoon as my partner and I watched a snail eating. The acid we had taken had let us become completely engaged in the moment, we were transfixed by the beauty of this tiny creature. On another occasion (using STP and LSD combined) I witnessed a friend become a beautiful lion, while for him I became a hawk. In a later trip we were both able to transform into these 'power animals' and experience some of their atavistic power. Perhaps for me the most lucid experience was during my second acid trip, the first I had ever taken with another person. As clouds covered the full moon I saw a wolf. Not a clear hallucination but more than just a fleeting impression. For a whole variety of reasons this encounter had personal meaning for me (not least of which was that my tripping companion's family name means 'wolf'). I could hear the sounds of the creature's breathing and its padding along the wall beside me. Rather than feeling fear I was greatly encouraged, and even reassured by the creature's presence. As it sniffed around us the acid really started kicking in and my friend and I were left 'like giants moving upon the land', far out into the liminal state but protected (though we were in the centre of a city) by our wolf ally.

Here is an American anthropologist's account about his transformation into a wild animal;

> At about the same instant I found myself before a full-length mirror and, looking into it, was confronted by a huge, magnificent specimen of a tiger! Simultaneously, I think, with my perception

of this image, I became aware of my tiger's body...I was *in* this body, and *felt* this body as I never have been in or felt my own. Yet even with what seemed my complete immersion in my tigerness, I did retain some infinitesimal human awareness...Would I have appeared to an observer to resemble in any way a tiger? Somehow I think the answer to that is 'Yes'. But probably, I now feel obliged to add, I would only have looked like a silly anthropologist, 'out of his skull' on hallucinogens, foolishly crawling around on the floor and making idiotic noises[187]

As ever the materialism of western culture, rather than the usual devil of dualism, is responsible for the witness being compelled to cross-examine himself to the point where his account is reduced to being 'a lie'. This approach is quite different in some other cultures, where to be able to really understand culture it is necessary to step outside it.

...those who wished to come to know the essence of culture needed to go out into the wilderness. Only there could they discover their everyday nature which was familiar to them and yet unknown. At the height of the Middle Ages, Geoffrey of Monmouth wrote an account of the life of Merlin in the forests of Caledonia; Yvain, Lancelot, Tristan left culture behind to eat raw meat of animals, and to become mad in the wilderness, 'the realm from which no stranger ever returned'. Only having become wild could they rise to the rank of knight. Following the same path, the Tungus shaman runs out into the wilderness, or his 'soul' travels down the kin river, the *mumangi chokto bira*, the 'watery river path', to the spirits of the ancestors. His tambourine acts as his companion, assuming the shape of an eider goose or of a pike, and he uses the drumstick as a rudder. Finally, he reaches the 'shaman tree of his clan'. Its roots reach into the lower world, its top stretches to the upper world, and humans live around the middle section of its trunk. *Ijäkyl*, the 'animal mother of the shaman', lies among the roots. She swallows the shaman's soul and gives birth to it in animal shape. From that day forward, the shaman possesses 'another side' of his person, his 'animal part' (*chargi*), which lives out in the *taiga* in a lonely tree.[188]

Sometimes animal/human interactions whilst tripping are less about transformation than they are about communion or identification. A friend told me how, while using psychedelics in Richmond park, London, he saw a huge king stag. The beast was sitting in the centre of the field as if the very space were radiating out of him. My friend then experienced a tremendous sense of kinship with the animal, an inner recognition of its power and nobility and found himself standing in a posture that 'resembled the hind leg of the creature'. My friend found the sense of being both of (in his posture) and impressed by the stag (as a 'royal beast') a powerful and illumining experience.

Oliver Sacks relates a story in *The Man who Mistook His Wife for a Hat* of a young medical student who, after using amphetamines, was propelled into the sensory perspective of a dog. He developed for a period of a few days, hyperacute smell and lived for a short time in a world in which this atavistic power had surfaced in his consciousness.

Other drugs can also unlock these changes in perception of form. Antonio Melechi, writing in *Fortean Times* on kinaesthesia, that is 'the body's awareness of its own *schema*';

> Volunteers under the influence of mescaline would often report feeling themselves physically transformed when subjected to different sensations. 'The barking of a dog' revealed one volunteer, 'vibrated through my right foot. This was so distinct that I thought it necessary to identify the dog with my right foot.' This sense of bodily mutation was echoed by other volunteers who reported feeling themselves becoming objects they touched or viewed."[189] Of course these transformations may not always be into animals, they can also be into objects or plants. Here is an account from someone experimenting with the powerful psychedelic plant *Salvia divinorum*, reported in *The Entheogen Review*;

"...five minutes of uncontrollable laughter, followed by visions 'similar to those in fantasy paintings or ancient oriental palaces: the Alhambra of Grenada. A large, almost endless empty hall with beautiful arches and hundreds of columns: all in a strange, gloomy, blue-gray light with colors of deep magic and majesty.'

This person later went on to feel as if he'd become a tree, similar to an oak. He experienced his bark as a sense organ, and remarked, 'while it was happening I had no doubt that a tree feels that way.'[190]

## Other Voices

Telepathy of one sort or another is without doubt one of the most commonly experienced phenomena during drug experiences. This often manifests itself between those who have taken the same drug but can, though more rarely in my experience, emerge between the person who is stoned and a straight individual. The experience of knowing what your companion is thinking when under the influence of psychedelics is so common place as to be rarely remarked upon. For some cultures the power of telepathic communication which a drug can induce is seen as a vital and powerful part of its action. The tribal preparation ayahuasca has marked telepathic properties for those who take it together. So much so that when one active chemical ingredient was first isolated from the brew it was named *telepathin*.

Drugs can also facilitate translation of meaning across different languages. A simple example of this from my own experience is the first time that I got really stoned on hashish. Myself and a friend were travelling and were camped outside for the night in southern France at the foot of cliff, overlooking the Mediterranean. A Frenchman happened past and, though we spoke little French and he not much English, we established that he would give us a smoke in return for some of the fish that we were cooking. Later that night, as we lay smoking on the rocks he told us about the bats that were circling overhead. Although I was unable to decipher his words, I could never-the-less make quite detailed sense of his soliloquy. Certainly my rudimentary knowledge of French helped, but the point was that the drug seemed to let meaning flow more easily. This may be simply due to the fact that I could relax and focus my attention on communication clues I could read (such as body language, French words with common Latin roots, tone of voice, etc.).

Serena Roney-Dougal, in her book *Where Science and Magic Meet,* suggests that the same chemicals that are stimulated by hallucinogenic drugs in the brain, might in some way be connected with psychic ability. She notes that much of the folklore we have concerning second sight can be read in neurochemical terms.

Certainly in terms of ancient and contemporary tribal cultures the 'messages' that a person might get during a drug experience may not be purely produced by the individual's own mind. They may come from ancestors, from other members of the group or indeed from non-human entities. In any case, although this is not to say that critical thought is absent with regard to these experiences, these cultures do not automatically assume that these messages either emerge from the person who 'hears' them, nor that they are without significance.

In terms of telepathic ability we might also consider the experience of the schizophrenic. Although these voices may come from the schizophrenic brain, they are clearly projected 'outwards' as apparently real, audible sounds. These voices may know things that the individual does not consciously have knowledge of (much like the type of knowledge that is accessible through hypnosis). The fact that we are continually enmeshed in a web of information 'speech' and meaning in our cultures (whether we are on drugs or not) means that it is hardly surprising that sometimes information can come to us in ways that we simply do not understand.[191]

We might think of telepathy as the externalised schizophrenic voices that express 'dark' sensory information. So although I 'know' how so-and-so feels I do so through subtle, subliminal, unconscious means. Therefore in order to express this knowledge to myself I externalise it as a 'telepathic voice' that tells me what I (apparently) am not aware of. It may also be true that telepathic abilities represent another method of shifting our real-yet-imaginary sense of 'I' from the realm of personal conscious knowledge, out into the field of some type of collective, cultural or super-sensory experience.[192]

Telepathic ability is featured in the use of San Pedro, as reported by anthropologist Douglas Sharon in *Flesh of the Gods;*

> ...first, a slight dizziness that one hardly notices. And then a great vision, a clearing of all faculties of the individual. It produces a slight numbness in the body and afterwards a tranquillity. And then comes a detachment, a type of visual force in the individual, inclusive of all senses; seeing, hearing, smelling, touching, etc. – all the senses, including the sixth sense, the telepathic sense of transmitting oneself across time and matter.[193]

In practice the idea of telepathy as a distinct supernatural power is too simplistic. Drug experiences can include all manner of sensory alterations and novel combinations. As well as receiving information apparently from another mind, one might also receive knowledge from the future. Drugs have long been used for divinatory purposes. Divination is, '...the art and science of discovering by organised intuition the past of an individual, their present situation and outlining possible courses of action and possible results of any given course.' [194]

The chronicler Gonzalvo Fernando d'Oviedo y Valdez wrote about the divinatory use of drugs by the Indians of Hispaniola, that they:

...have secret means of putting themselves in touch with spirits whenever they wished to predict the future...When the chief called one of those priests of the desert, this man came with two of his disciples, one of whom bore a vase filled with some mysterious drink...He drank the liquor which had been brought, and then began his conjurations, calling aloud on the spirits; and then, highly agitated and furious, he was shaken by the most violent movements...He then seemed to be plunged into a kind of ecstasy and to be suffering curious pains...When the priest calmed down, and while he lay senseless on the ground the chief, or some other, asked what they desired to know, and the spirit replied through the mouth of the inspired man in a manner perfectly exact.

Personally I have found that the tail end of MDMA intoxication is an ideal state in which to conduct tarot readings. Where the mind of the reader and that of the client can be relaxed and where symbolic and intuitive information can be sought and exchanged with remarkable ease.[195]

Lilly, in his experiments using LSD and sensory deprivation frequently found that the 'noise' created in the mind by LSD intoxication would often lead to 'random' neural effects becoming organised into information. From the 'white noise' of the mind, '...one can hear what one wants (or fears) to hear, human voices talking about one, or one's enemies discussing plans, etc.' But in the end the content of this information cannot always be neatly glossed over in terms of the individual mind 'making things up'. Lilly goes on to identify four possible sources for 'information received from 'outside'; '(1) inside one's own head; (2) from other beings, nonhuman; (3) from outer space intelligences; (4) from ESP with humans.'[196] There may well be other sources of information but the point for me is that through drug experience one can learn to dissolve the Self/Other boundary. This can then lead to the transmission of information which is, in our culture, 'supernatural'.[197]

## Magic Carpet Ride

A whole range of magical powers or, to use the yogic term, *siddhis* are accessible during or through sacred drug experience.

During one intoxicated experience I was able to pick up glowing coals and remain unharmed. Although I didn't think much about it at the time, after the experience (which was during a Midsummer ceremony) I realised that although 'I' had done it, the experience had in fact seemed to flow *through* me. In many cases where magical abilities are demonstrated, the individual often claims that he or she is 'a channel' through which divine grace, or magical power, or the spirit of the San Pedro (or whatever), flows.

Abilities which can come to magicians through the use of drugs can be tremendously varied. They include the ability to set objects alight by thought, the ability to make objects mysteriously appear, feats of 'psychic surgery' (for example when a shaman 'sucks out' a harmful 'magical dart' from a patient to cure illness)[198] and more. To the western mind those siddhis that we are most likely to believe in are those which we can see as being about control of the 'self'. For instance the ability to endure extreme temperature, to remain motionless for long periods, to cut the skin without loss of blood. We can accept our dominion of 'I' when it is located in the body and brain of the individual, yet we have no real idea of how this 'I' is in control in the first place. For other cultures, where 'I' is just a small part of my being, and can be located either within or without my physical form, magical abilities seem much less fanciful.

The drug experience can lead to the discovery of new abilities but this discovery rests upon being able to give up one's usual sense of 'I'. To have power, to have the siddhis of the chemical gnosis, is to let the universe flow through you. It is to let 'you' become bigger than your usual sense of mind and 'I'. These powers are erratic but shamanic rituals certainly seek to promote the conditions within which they can appear. The sacred use of drugs is one such condition.

Let me give a slightly less 'supernatural' example of this process of power 'flowing through'. A friend told me a story of how, when he was really stoned (and during a period in his life when he'd been experimenting extensively with LSD) he became an inspired mediator. He was able to non-violently intervene in a riotous dispute between festival goers and security guards. By a combination of actions and joking addresses he was able to defuse a dangerous situation. In his recollection the events happened *through* him. It was the drug experience that allowed the spirit of a 'joking Jesus freak' to emerge and win over both parties, averting serious violence.

## At the Sill of the Door

By suggesting that drug experience can give us access to 'supernatural' effects and powers I am not suggesting that the world is completely malleable. The paradox of drugs is the same as the paradox of magic - namely that the world can be influenced by the mind, but also that the mind is part of the world. Magical experiences, mystical insight, indeed much of human experience is capricious and unpredictable. Moreover, magical effects occur in the liminal sphere that drug experiences occupy. For example in a case of apparent telepathy it is often difficult to establish whether the 'intuition' felt is the result of 'dark' sensory activity, some effect of non-localised consciousness (shifting the location of one's sense of 'I' to occupy the thoughts of another person), or a change in our usual sequential sense of time or whatever. Psychic phenomena are not above investigation but it would be a mistake to think that, just because it is difficult to experimentally establish the repeatability of magical phenomena, they are simply the product of wishful thinking. Even with effects that are amenable to experimental analysis the effects of 'psi' are undoubtedly subtle. However so too are the effects of many other things that we accept as true.[199]

Today many writers who are interested in the existence of psychic phenomena seek the explanation for these things in terms of modern quantum physics.[200] The problem with this is that it assumes that the method of science is *a priori* correct and that 'extraordinary claims require extraordinary proof'; and that this proof can only be gleaned from the weird outer limits of the scientific discourse. This is an example of autistic thinking. Namely that the world can be categorised into discrete, objective units that can be understood in isolation from one another. Indeed the very existence of the scientific laboratory (whether it be the actual laboratory where rats run round mazes, or the theoretical laboratory of mathematical equations) presumes that we can isolate specific elements in the world and analyse them. Of course there have been many critiques of this practice, especially by post-modernist scholars.[201]

If we can alter the world then the world can alter us, since where we choose to place the dividing line between Self and Other is quite arbitrary. Although the shaman may wield magical powers, these powers are uncertain and come at the price of opening the Self (the sense of 'I') to the winds of change and transgression. The shaman is more sensitive to atmospheres, more exposed to the danger of madness (i.e. transgressing and being unable to make the shamanic return). Even the most powerful magician, the greatest martial artist, the most gifted psychic is not in absolute control of their world. I stress this point because there is a horrible tendency on the part of new age writers to suggest that the universe is entirely the product of our minds. The argument is that misfortune is, in effect, brought on ourselves and that we can have complete dominion over the world through nothing more elaborate than pseudo-mystical positive thinking.[202]

Although the root of the word magic means 'power' this is not necessarily power which flows from the individual out into the world. I feel that the magician/shaman is better thought of as the mediator between the worlds of humans and of the gods. The magician aims to enter, use and explore the liminal world, to learn and to change. In this sense taking intelligent control of our life means to become a magician, but this also requires letting go of established values and points of reference. As writers such as the witch Starhawk have pointed out, power (whether magical or otherwise) is as much something that flows through us, that is allied with us, as much as it is imposed by us.[203]

## The Second Twilight

Most tribal cultures populate the universe with a vast array of invisible beings. In the west we also have a rich tradition of folklore and demonology which describes this invisible world. In one sense this practice is continued by modern people. We are prepared to imagine invisible forces (such as gravity, electro-magnetism and the 'particulate personifications' of these forces as quarks, atoms, waves, neutrinos etc.). Yet materialist culture is incredulous of the idea that, parallel to the visible realm, there is a whole supernatural order of ghosts, spirits, elementals and gods. This is an understandable reaction given the fact that western culture has only just wrestled itself away from the idea that there is an invisible god controlling things, and this god has a moral agenda which the priesthood had the sole right to interpret.

I believe that much of the western reading of shamanic entities (and for that matter our modern appreciation of demons in the sense that

Descartes or medieval magicians used the term) is based on much misguided interpretation. It is biased less toward trying to understand another model of the world, than it is created in order to defend the assumptions of our current world view. I have argued that it is quite possible for the world to exist as an objective fact and for the mind to be an interacting thing of a different order of being. There really isn't a problem if we learn to accept the paradox that the shaman can fly and yet that her body remains on the earth, no more than an intelligent modern person is supposed to have difficulty grasping that light is a wave and a particle.

The magical manifestations of drug experience can certainly include interacting with beings that have the appearance of external, real, intelligent entities.[204] Certainly the DMT experience, with its commonplace visions of fairies or aliens, can provide a gateway to this invisible realm.

So are these entities independent, conscious beings or simply 'figments of our imagination'? To answer this we have to remember that believing something is conscious depends very much on empathy, perspective and where we choose to draw the arbitrary line between Self/Other. For example if you are driving along a motorway and see cars waiting to join the flow of traffic you may well assume that each car contains a conscious, thinking human being, even if you cannot see them behind the wheel. If you looked at the motorway from the air, you would see a whole host of metal boxes, perhaps charging into the city in the early hours and exiting in the evening. Now step back further. Imagine that you are so far away that all you see is a series of dots, tiny somethings moving along defined routes. Of course from this perspective the idea that each car's movement is the result of a thinking, feeling human being gets progressively lost. Eventually all we are left to deal with is the movement of 'car particles' which, we might imagine are being motivated by all sorts of external 'laws'. So when we look at cells flowing through veins we tend to see them as being subjects of external forces (capillary action, clotting, cardiac rhythm). Of course there is nothing wrong with considering these external forces, any more than it would be inappropriate to analyse the movement of cars into cities in terms of economic factors or the history of transport infrastructures. Even so it is equally acceptable, in my view, to consider the consciousness of the drivers themselves (otherwise why bother with emotive anti-speeding campaigns and roadside billboards?).

Of course many cultures attribute a spirit to the material basis of things, especially if those things are powerful drugs (in much the same way that interactionalists would attribute the existence of a spirit or mind that is paired to the physical structure of the brain). Perhaps even for modern people the spirit of some drugs is so potent that the material basis of the drug is only part of its story. There is, for instance, the curious story of how LSD's psychedelic power was discovered. Here is Hofmann's account from *LSD My Problem Child*:

And yet I could not forget the relatively uninteresting LSD-25. A peculiar presentiment - the feeling that this substance could possess properties other than those established in the first investigations - induced me, five years after the first synthesis, to produce LSD-25 once again so that a sample could be given to the pharmacological department for further tests. This was quite unusual; experimental substances, as a rule, were definitely stricken from the research program if once found to be lacking in pharmacological interest.

Perhaps the 'spirit of LSD' spoke to Hofmann? We could of course say Hofmann's feelings were 'after the fact' but, as they say, just because one can fake an orgasm doesn't mean they don't happen.

The magical traditions and the shamanic complex recognise a drug as having its own spirit. Drug experience can allow us to experience that spirit as it relates to us, and may perhaps provide a glimpse of the other denizens of the Other which our science ignores.

# Break on Through: the experience of drugs

## Right Here, Right Now

In this section I'm going to examine a few specific drugs more closely. Of course the effects that I ascribe to a given material are, in part, the result of personal and cultural factors. Indeed the placebo effect, and cultural expectations play a vital role in understanding the history of the LSD experience in particular. So, though for the sake of simplicity I say 'ecstasy does such-and-such', I clearly recognise the subjectivity and cultural dependence of my statements. Paradoxically, I have also discovered a number of quite specific effects of some of the drugs that I examine below. Although much of my evidence is anecdotal I believe that the paradoxical effects of drug experience are demonstrated by the accounts I have collected; by the simultaneous facts that a) the experience of a given drug can differ widely and b) that very specific effects can be shared.

I have included a few of the more exotic drug materials in this section, but I have concentrated my attention on those drugs that are commonly available in the west. The reason for this is that I want to stress that all the transcendent, transgressive experience we need (in terms of drug experience) is available right here and now. The idea that, at the borders of ethnopharmacology, there is a new synthetic, or ancient brew that is the new saviour chemical is a big mistake. Certainly there are lots of exotic and rare drugs out there that are worth exploring and I genuinely admire chemists like Alexander Shulgin and those intrepid 'psychonauts' who spend their time trying to discover and explore new drugs.

Obviously my own relationships with various drugs is in a continuous process of change, what I write about a given drug today could change dramatically tomorrow. This is especially true (for me) of the hallucinogenic drugs, which, by their very nature, are easy to imagine as having moods and intentions. The following might be thought of as a broad description of how the spirits[205] of these drugs appear.

I would recommend that readers interested in exploring one or more of these substances start by searching the internet through which a vast array of drug-oriented information may be obtained.

## Δ9-THC - Cannabis

Cannabis is extremely responsive to set and setting. In part the various sensations experienced when using cannabis may be due to the many different situations in which the drug is commonly employed. The use of cannabis across the globe is widespread and commonplace. This means that the same user, using roughly the same dosage, may have been exposed to the cannabis effect at work, whilst relaxing on holiday, in bed with a lover or in a number of other solitary or social situations.

Variations of the experience are also determined by dosage and the method of administration. Generally speaking smoking the flowers of the plant is a much more gentle experience that eating quantities of the resin. The resin is particularly potent if it has first been dissolved into fat (as per the traditional bhang lassi – cannabis yoghurt drink – of Indian culture) which assists absorption in the stomach.

The range and depth of cannabis effects serves to show, quite clearly, how one drug material can participate in a wide range of drug experiences. It can produce states of lethargy and sleep or activity and talkativeness. Internally the experience can range from intense psychedelic changes in perception, through elation to the depths of dark paranoia. Cannabis intoxication can lead to marvellous, often humorous and frequently meandering story telling. As the fibre of the plant itself is ideal for weaving and rope making, so in language cannabis helps us spin hilarious stories, punctuated by endless tangents and deviations. Cannabis can gently open up the structure of spoken language and lead to the type of free association often sought by psychotherapy. Cannabis is also called 'wisdom weed' and can seem to propel the mind at great speed so that the paradoxes, refutations and internal contradictions (Derrida's trace) can be seen in any idea or statement. This can lead to fun, to inspiration and to the ability to think things out, at 'high speed' from a number of different and (usually) mutually incompatible perspectives.

The experience of cannabis is, for many people, very much a learnt response. To some degree this is true of all drugs. Our bodies initially register that this is a foreign, perhaps mildly 'toxic'[206] substance. Vomiting, general disorientation, nervous physical and psychological responses are common in the initial engagement with many drugs ('depressants' such as alcohol, tobacco, cannabis and opium being the most common materials that seem to go through this phase of relationship with the user). For me it took some years of experimenting with dope to finally 'get it', and 'work out' how to get stoned.[207] Prior to getting properly stoned for the first time, generally all I would experience from cannabis was a general spinning, light-headed sensation, often nausea, and occasionally vomiting. Learning to get stoned, to successfully move one's mind set, sense of self or 'point of assemblage'[208] into 'hash space', takes practice. The same is true, as McKenna and others have pointed out, with developing any type of 'taste for', whether the material is psychedelics, curry or wine.

Shamanism might be thought of as the ability to know, enter, explore and return from drug states. In the case of cannabis, as with so many other drugs, use and experience deepen one's appreciation for, and potential range of experiences within the drug state.

## LSD

The chemical structure of LSD is very similar to that of serotonin and it is generally assumed that the LSD experience is caused by it interacting in some way with this neurochemical system. The exact way that this takes place is still disputed (as demonstrated by Steve Finney who provides an excellent overview of the state of pharmacological research into LSD).[209]

Tolerance to LSD develops very quickly in humans, so much so that it has been called an 'anti-addictive' drug. After taking LSD, an identical dose taken a few days later is likely to produce little or no effect. Increasing the dose may generate a psychedelic experience but something of the 'freshness' of the trip is dulled. Individual tolerance varies. Some users are happy leaving seven days between trips in order for each dose to have a full effect. Others (myself included) prefer to leave at least 30 days. In this respect the blurred line between psychological and pharmacological is again apparent. Although one might have, chemically, returned to zero physiological tolerance after a trip, one might not have returned to zero psychological tolerance. The longer the gap between trips the more powerful each one is likely to be, as the individual has more time to withdraw from the drug experience (making the 'shamanic return') and build it into an everyday rational framework.

The speed at which LSD works can also vary dramatically. Generally between 30 minutes and 1 hour is thought to be the average time before the first sensations of the drug are felt if it is taken orally. (However, as mentioned above, I have experienced 'coming up' on a trip within 15 minutes.)

A friend, who is an astrologer, told me some years ago that he felt that LSD should be described as being under the rulership of Pluto.[210] Pluto in astrology, as in classical myth, is the ruler of the underworld, the realm of the unconscious mind. Moreover the symbol of Pluto stands for the explosive moment of transgression, the extreme cusp of death and rebirth. The images called to mind are of the moment when the sperm penetrates the ovum and explodes its genetic information into the egg cell, or the fusion reaction which begins a star's ignition.

For me LSD is certainly a Plutonian drug – in terms of pure quantity it is one of the most powerful drugs known and its essential psychedelic effect is *'solve et coagula'*, to break the world up, to smash it into fragments of visual distortion and strange meaning. And then, to recombine it. To merge previously irreconcilable elements of the world together, to make one see the infinite in the finite, to sense that one is part of a great cosmic whole.[211] The fact that, microgram for microgram, LSD is the most powerful psychedelic reiterates this 'atomic' symbolism of astrology.[212] Just a tiny amount of LSD can rip your universe apart with awesome consequences.[213] It can fuse experience together in a mystical oneness and, perhaps most important, it can generate both of these experiences simultaneously.

LSD can be its own ritual. Each LSD experience has the definite character of a journey, a 'trip', a ritual, an adventure. As many LSD users will wryly tell you, one of the oddest effects of LSD is that weird things often happen on it. It is common for someone who is talking about their LSD experiences to say something along the lines of 'sure, I know I was on acid but I'm sure that such-and-such *really* happened'. The weird event in question can vary from the urbane (such as going into a pub and seeing a group of drinkers who, for some reason, are dressed as clowns), through to the thoroughly mysterious (seeing UFOs, being capable of superhuman feats and so on). The 'reality' or 'intra-subjectivity' of these events is of less importance than the very fact that they are reported. LSD shakes up the boundaries of the world so much that categories like real/imaginary, true/false become destabilised.

Historically LSD demonstrates how drug lore can be just as important in shaping drug experience as any chemical concoction in itself. Until the 1960s the LSD experience was pretty much considered one phenomena. Although trips could include 'easy' or 'difficult', and contain different points of focus, acid was essentially thought of as a variable but specific type of drug experience. Your trip might well be *your* trip but it was essentially just a personal view of the acid experience. This situation changed as a result of two interactive factors. The first was the concerted campaign on the part of a number of discourses (most obvious in their manifestation as 'the media') to spread scare stories about the drug. As Bruce Eisner writes 'Expectations about the LSD experience strongly influence the nature of the experience…Prior to 1962, there were very few negative experiences reported by those who experienced LSD.'[214] A feedback loop was set up in drug culture. In trying to understand stories about widely differing experiences due to the action of the one drug (ranging from the old chestnut of crazed college youths jumping out of fifth story windows, to the idea that LSD could cause genetic damage)[215] people sought the answer in the chemical composition of the drug. When the underground chemist Owsley was synthesising LSD in the United States he decided to colour code different batches. Although chemically the dye was inert the different colours of acid quickly developed different reputations.[216] Red acid was said to be more intense, green coloured acid more mellow, purple more spiritual and so on.

LSD is a powerful drug, active at doses as low as 50 micrograms. Therefore having gone to the bother of making the clandestine chemical, it is hardly necessary to adulterate it. As Bruce Eisner, writing in High Times in 1977 observed '… there is rarely speed or strychnine in street acid. The most common additive is PCP (phencyclidine, or Serylan, an animal tranquilliser that causes hallucinogenic delirium reactions), which is also present when street acid is mislabelled "mescaline" or "psilocybin".'[217] Although there certainly are impurities in street acid today the major variable in the effect of the trip (from a chemical perspective) is the dose. As Hofmann himself pointed, out LSD is highly susceptible to chemical degradation by light and oxidising agents. LSD is liquid at room temperature (hence the wise precaution of keeping it in the refrigerator) and so a blotter (the most common packaging for street LSD) will lose it potency over time depending on the conditions in which it is kept.

The LSD molecule itself comes in the form of four basic variations, only one of which is the powerful psychedelic that people generally mean when they talk about LSD. The other forms of LSD may be present as impurities but are likely simply to reduce the effectiveness of their active counterpart.[218]

In short, although acid may have been 'better in the old days' (assuming your old days were during the period of LSD's legality) impurities are an inevitable but fairly inconsequential part of the street acid experience. The variation of acid experience is far more likely to be influenced by set and setting and dosage, than it is by whether the acid is 'clean' or not.[219]

Considering its powerful destruction of the boundaries between Self and Other, LSD is remarkable as Albert Hofmann recognises in *LSD My Problem Child*:

> What seemed even more significant [than the extremely low dose at which LSD is active] was that I could remember the experience of LSD inebriation in every detail. This could only mean that the conscious recording function was not interrupted, even in the climax of the LSD experience, despite the profound breakdown of the normal worldview. For the entire duration of the experiment, I had even been aware of participating in an experiment, but despite this recognition of my condition, I could not, with every exertion of my will, shake off the LSD world. Everything was experienced as completely real, as alarming reality; alarming, because the picture of the other, familiar everyday reality was still fully preserved in the memory for comparison.

Because the experience of LSD does not generally include the loss of memory (which is a common feature in drug experiences reached with solanaceous plants such as nightshade) it can be directly linked back to the world. This is especially true if the shamanic return is managed well. For this reason LSD (in common with psychedelics such as mescaline and psilocybin) has powerful potential as an aid to psychotherapy. Indeed studies before and after the prohibition of LSD have shown that, in the hands of an experienced and sensitive therapist (or shaman, or magician) acid can be a great aid to mental healing.[220]

The experience of 'peaking' on acid can put you utterly in the realm of 'madness', yet the experience can still be apprehended and, in some sense, remembered. A peak moment of acid happens outside of language, it is something which we can remember afterwards but is itself virtually inexpressible. Of course this does not only go for acid but for most types of numinous experience. One of the advantages of acid is that it puts the body under little stress in getting to the numinous peak (unlike, say fasting), however the very fact of this means that it may be a difficult experience for someone who comes to it without prior training in altered states of consciousness. Naturally most people who enjoy acid, even if they have never explored meditation, ritual or other spiritual practices, can cope admirably with it. We should not assume that 'training in altered states' should come from an external teacher. After all who was it that initiated the first shaman and gave her the first magical brew to drink?

Perhaps because of its astrologically Plutonian nature (or perhaps for historical reasons as a 'swinging sixties' drug), LSD has a great affinity with that other powerful boundary dissolving experience, sex. Although some people report ecstatic sexuality on LSD, most users find that they are somewhat less liable to sexual arousal simply because the drug experience itself is so powerful. Any additional stimulus is hard to focus on and sequential acts become fragmented and fail to hold one's attention in the usual way. Many people, however, in my experience find that they feel an increase in sexual arousal after the trip has ended. In part this might be thought of as both a fitting means for expressing the insights of LSD as well as a method of 'grounding' the Self in the physical soma.

There are accounts of women conceiving on LSD and there is perhaps some evidence that LSD might well stimulate ovulation (even at quite unlikely points in an individual's menstrual cycle).[221]

It is also quite common for people to want to wash, often to bathe, after acid. Again in part this may be a simple relaxing, 'grounding' practice. It may also be thought of as a kind of re-baptism into the world and made into a conscious part of the ritual of transgression. For some people the desire to bathe is because acid leaves them feeling physically dirty. In part this may be due to the strange but subtle tactile hallucinations that LSD creates, sometimes making surfaces (including one's own skin) feeling dusty or greasy.

## Magic Mushrooms

There are a number of different psychedelic mushrooms that are employed around the world, from 'blue meanies' in Australia, through to the infamous fly agaric[222] of north-western Europe. Different mushrooms contain different active drugs but the most common are tryptamine based hallucinogens of which psilocin and psilocybin are the most usual.

Whilst mushroom trips may be as powerful (particularly at reasonably large doses) as LSD, most users report a sense that mushrooms are 'easier to deal with'. Mushroom trips often feel 'earthier', less like the clinical cutting open of the mind that acid is apt to do, they are generally gentler and contain less of the sense of profound strangeness that LSD provokes. Depending on circumstances the mushroom experience can provoke an outpouring of emotions, ranging (sometimes in literally minutes) from uncontrolled weeping to giggling laughter. Famously mushrooms, like MDMA, sometimes provoke what psychologists call 'pressure of speech'. There can be a strong desire to talk. Speech can become at times profound, at other times tied into knots (although there is usually less of the rambling that comes with smoking hashish). Words often shift their meaning and often both the speaker and listener will derive some hitherto unforeseen interpretation. In some cultures magic mushrooms are significantly linked to speaking as a magical act. Henry Munn writes of the use of *Psilocybe mexicana*, which is traditionally used by the Mazatex Indians of Mexico. In this context the shaman, often along with other members of the community, ingest the mushrooms. The mushrooms then speak through the shaman, sometimes as poetry, often as sung chants. 'Language is an ecstatic activity of signification. Intoxicated by the mushrooms, the fluency, the ease, the aptness of expression one becomes capable of are such that one is astounded by the words that issue forth.'[223]

The sense of the 'rightness of words', of their multifaceted meaning and their profundity, was certainly my experience when, around February 1998 I took part in an American Indian style ritual. The ritual itself was based around the format of the Native American peyote ceremony. But rather than take peyote, myself and around 34 other people, consumed magic mushrooms. Although I did not speak, I was able to hear a number of other people doing so during the course of the ritual. Whatever was said was subject to two, normally mutually exclusive phenomena. Firstly that what was said was 'just right', apt and poetically perfect. Secondly, that whatever was said was subject to a multiplicity of meanings and interpretations and I (and others) felt immediately aware of this.

These observations back up Terence McKenna's claim that '…human language may have arisen when primate organizational potential was synergized by plant hallucinogens. The psychedelic experience inspired us to true self-reflective thought in the first place and then further inspired us to communicate our thoughts about it.' Whilst I feel that McKenna's argument does have its faults he may certainly have identified an important link between drug experience and humanity within the context of an evolutionary model of how we came to be. He goes on to point out that 'Psilocybin specifically activates the areas of the brain concerned with processing signals. A common occurrence with psilocybin intoxication is spontaneous outbursts of poetry and other vocal activity…Researchers familiar with the territory agree that psilocybin has a profoundly catalytic effect on the linguistic impulse.'[224]

Mushrooms can also provoke a wonderful range of visual changes in the world. LSD, even at quite high doses need not produce the kind of visuals associated with mushrooms. In my own experience at the 'mushroom 'peyote' ceremony' I was aware that the inside of the tepee canvas was covered in what looked like faint watermarks of graphically stylised art, ancient Egyptian or perhaps Mayan in style. The logs on the central fire, as the bark was burning away from the timber, were covered in strange unreadable runes.[225]

The presence of graphic imagery in the mushroom experience is recounted by Albert Hofmann in the following extract from his book *LSD My Problem Child*:

> Mrs. Li Gelpke, an artist, also participated in this series of investigations, taking three self-experiments with LSD and psilocybin. The artist wrote of the drawing she made during the experiment:
>
> *Nothing on this page is consciously fashioned. While I worked on it, the memory (of the experience under psilocybin) was again reality, and led me at every stroke. For that reason the picture is as many-layered as this memory, and the figure at the lower right is really the captive of its dream.... When books about Mexican art came into my hands three weeks later, I again found the motifs of my visions there with a sudden start....*
>
> I have also mentioned the occurrence of Mexican motifs in

psilocybin inebriation during my first self experiment with dried Psilocybe mexicana mushrooms, as was described in the section on the chemical investigation of these mushrooms. The same phenomenon has also struck R. Gordon Wasson. Proceeding from such observations, he has advanced the conjecture that ancient Mexican art could have been influenced by visionary images, as they appear in mushroom inebriation.[226]

Although the exact potency of a given mushroom can vary, one of the advantages of mushrooms is that just a little (or a few, perhaps ten in the case of European psilocybin) can be taken. This can provide either a gentle buzz for recreational purposes or can be used for the novice to ease their way into the territory of psychedelics. McKenna and others (perhaps drawing on the traditions of native peoples such as the Mazatex Indians) recommend that large doses are best taken in total darkness. This should be determined by one's own preference and experience. Certainly the practice of harvesting them fresh and eating 'on the hoof' can be a rewarding way to enjoy the great outdoors.

## DMT & Ayahuasca

As each drug is absorbed into western culture it tends to go through a stage where the most remarkable claims are made for it. In the case of Dimethyltryptamine (DMT) the story told is that it allows the user to enter into another, parallel universe.

Chemically synthesised DMT is usually smoked since the drug in this form is inactive if taken orally. The exception to this rule is if it is combined with MAO inhibitors. The orally active form of DMT usually forms part of the hallucinogenic brew ayahuasca.[227]

When smoked DMT precipitates the user into a profound psychedelic state. The onset of the drug's effects happen within a matter of seconds and peak between 5 to 15 minutes. There is then a gradual tailing off with the 'baseline' (i.e. 'normal' state) being reached after about half an hour. As already mentioned DMT may be implicated in spontaneous drug experiences, particularly since, at a suitable dose, the effect of the drug is to propel the user into 'hyperspace', a hallucinogenic realm which, many people report, comes complete with apparently external entities which have a 'machine like' or sometimes elfish or fairy quality about them.

Although by no means all users have discovered this realm of discarnate beings there does seem to be a fairly high correlation between different accounts about what lies beyond the lower dose, intense initial psychedelic visions that DMT provokes.

The initial DMT intoxication often includes the presence of strange audio hallucinations, sometimes a buzzing of the type one hears before fainting, sometimes the sound of a 'membrane' ripping or a 'carrier wave' tone. Many of these have interesting parallels with the sounds that are heard as the occult psycho-sexual energy of *kundalini* (the 'fire snake') is raised in yogic practice.[228]

Terence McKenna is perhaps the most well known writer concerned with DMT, and the internet is full of sites which collate the information from different magicians who have attempted this dramatic psychedelic. The implications of the presence of what McKenna calls 'the tykes' in the DMT vision has spawned a whole host of theories. Perhaps most interesting is the very fact that DMT literally seems to unlock the invisible realm that shamans have long claimed exists parallel, connected, yet invisible to our reality. A sample of some of these speculations is discussed by Peter Meyer:

(i) There are no alien entities at all; it's merely subjective hallucination. The DMT state may be interesting, even extremely interesting, but really there are no independently existing alien entities to be found.

(ii) DMT provides access to a parallel or higher dimension, a truly alternate reality which is, in fact, inhabited by independently existing intelligent entities forming (in the words of Terence McKenna) 'an ecology of souls.'

(iii) DMT allows awareness of processes at a cellular or even atomic level. DMT smokers are tapping into the network of cells in the brain or even into communication among molecules themselves. It might even be an awareness of quantum mechanical processes at the atomic or subatomic level.

(iv) DMT is, perhaps, a neurotransmitter in reptilian brains and in the older, reptilian parts of mammalian brains. Flooding the human brain with DMT causes the older reptilian parts of the brain to dominate consciousness, resulting in a state of awareness which appears totally alien (and sometimes very frightening) to the everyday monkey mind.

(v) A non-human intelligent species created humans by genetic modification of existing primate stock then retreated, leaving behind biochemical methods for contacting them. The psychedelic tryptamines are chemical keys that activate certain programs in the human brain that were placed there intentionally by this alien species.

(vi) The realm to which DMT provides access is the world of the dead. The entities experienced are the souls, or personalities, of the departed, which retain some kind of life and ability to communicate. The realm of dead souls, commonly accepted by cultures and societies other than that of the modern West, is now accessible using DMT.

(vii) The entities experienced are beings from another time who have succeeded in mastering the art of time travel, not in a way which allows materialization but in a way which allows them to communicate with conscious beings such as ourselves.

(viii) The entities are probes from an extraterrestrial or an extradimensional species, sent out to make contact with organisms such as ourselves who are able to manipulate their nervous systems in a way which allows communication to take place.

These hypotheses can be expanded and are, of course, vulnerable to objections. No doubt other hypotheses are possible. These matters will not be resolved until we have more data with which to test these and other hypotheses.[229]

Although the break-neck speed and profound otherworldlyness of DMT can be frightening, the DMT experience can seem to be curiously lacking (or perhaps 'outside') the emotional content of other psychedelics. With smoked DMT the experience is often compared to watching a film.

As with the DMT elves (and to a lesser degree with the graphic motifs and 'language centred' imagery of psilocybin mushrooms) there seems to be a remarkable consistency with ayahuasca visions. Of course this may (to a greater or lesser degree) be due to users simply knowing what to expect. Ayahuasca hallucinations tend to be more mythical and enveloping than LSD ones and there is a more direct sense of having entered another realm. Jaguars and other large cats, dragons and snakes and often flying machines (frequently UFOs) are reported. For many users there may be a period of trauma or even terror where they have to 'fight' with beings that appear, often in the form of snakes.

It seems that ayahuasaca stands somewhere between LSD (where the hallucinations 'grow out of the world' and where memory remains unimpaired) and Datura (where the Self may be completely enveloped in a fantastic realm and no sense of 'tripping' is recalled). Since ayahuasca is a complex pharmacological preparation the variable of 'substance' might be radically different in two different experiments. Generally it seems traditional shamans will have their own preferred recipe.

To date ayahuasca use remains legal in a Brazil and it is increasingly finding its way into 'new age' style shamanic Christian movements (some of which have surfaced in Europe).

# Ecstasy

The memory of taking a good hit of ecstasy for the first time is like the memory of falling in love. MDMA has been called an empathogen in that it promotes empathic feelings. This drug, perhaps more than any other, has profoundly changed the face of the 20$^{th}$ century.

So what does 'E' feel like? Being able to talk, feeling lucid but relaxed, able to express even fears and anxieties and feeling 'all right'. Being able to let your body flow and move, to become carried away by the music, to become gloriously entranced by the lights. To smile at people on the dance floor whom you've never met, to share that secret sense of chemical joy. To watch the city lights blur gently as you relax into the comfort of the taxi home. To cuddle your lover in bed, letting your mind wander softly through the reverie of thought before sleep.

Of course individual reactions can widely vary and pills are not without a whole range and depth of effects. Depending on set, setting, dose and the actual content of the pill[230] the E experience can be subtle, beautiful, depressing or even scary.[231] Though one benefit of MDMA is that its general effects are quite reliable. The emotional barriers of the self become relaxed. It calms the mind and body and yet, paradoxically, stimulates speech, and can make intense physical activity such as dancing, absorbingly pleasurable.

In *MDMA - The Ecstasy Story,* under the title 'Paradoxical Effects' Eisner writes:

> During many Ecstasy sessions, there comes a moment of calm, of complete stillness, which some meditators have compared to the headspace achieved during the practice of meditation. Because MDMA is a modification of amphetamine, it is this stillness which drug researchers pointed to when they suggested the class of drugs represented by MDMA and MDA as having a "paradoxical effect". When someone takes an ordinary amphetamine such as dexedrine or methedrine, they most usually become agitated, restless and driven. Yet this class of amphetamine derivatives - oddly, paradoxically - brings a peaceful, relaxed, calm state upon the mind and body.

MDMA has been called an 'entactogen' meaning to 'touch within'. The term was coined by David Nichols, of the Department of Medicinal Chemistry of Purdue University, USA. Thus MDMA does not only serve to facilitate interpersonal communication (as an empathogen – i.e. an aid to empathy) but also (Eisner) '...transformation of the inner *psyche* - [and therefore] has uses in therapy and problem solving, meditation, self-actualisation, and creativity.' [232]

As well as the 'talk centred' opportunity for processing, transgressing and being creative that MDMA affords, dancing whilst under the influence of ecstasy can be a profound meditation. The ease with which physical movement comes can free the mind, allowing it to become both involved and relaxed within the physical dance. For what seems like long periods of time the mind can focus on the clubland lights, the sensations of the music or simply its own state of awareness. Nicholas Saunders comments on this interpretation of ecstasy dance as meditation. He quotes a Soto Zen monk who says that;

> 'Drugs do not go with meditation', but adds 'Meditation goes

wonderfully with drugs'. There is no contradiction; although drugs like MDMA may disturb acquired patterns of meditation, it is easy to meditate while under their influence. 'Being still when taking MDMA helps you to *know* how to sit, it provides you with experiential knowledge.' But is it a good way to learn? 'It is like a medicine. If we look at the state of our own minds and the planet, we should be grateful for any means that can help. However, like any good medicine, it can be misused.'

Although some users are able to use MDMA whilst motionless and seated in a meditative posture, meditation does not necessarily imply stillness of the body. Saunders goes on to quote a Rinzai Zen monk who accepted Saunders' invite to a party:

> ...eventually his face glowed and he announced 'This is meditation - to be truly in the moment and not in your head!' He later explained that the object of meditation was to cease the internal dialogue and yet be fully aware of what was happening, and that is exactly what the dancers were doing.
>
> Next morning he said he had had a revelation; his school of Zen concentrated too much on contraction such as disciplined meditation, but what was really needed by most students was the opposite, to let go and expand in the way he had just witnessed at the party. 'I can only hope that I will live long enough for the law to be changed so I am able to use Ecstasy for teaching' he said. A year later he was still as enthusiastic.

My partner and a friend gave me the opportunity to see, in dramatic terms, the paradoxical similarity yet divergent nature of drug experience, specifically in terms of ecstasy. Both reported that, during some MDMA experiences they hallucinated 'spectacles' being worn by everyone. It is paradoxical that one drug (which can certainly muster a whole range of different effects given different set, setting and substance variables) can come up with the exact same hallucination, for two different individuals, on a regular basis. Such a specific and idiosyncratic effect (both parties showed an evident amazement at meeting another person who shared their own peculiar effect from MDMA) demonstrates again how drug experience can be both different *and* shared.

Commonly people who are new to experimenting with ecstasy will dream about coming up (this has been reported to me by a number of users). This is especially common after the first few doses, especially if these occur within a reasonably short space of time. Once again this effect can be deconstructed in psychological or psychoanalytic terms. Otherwise we might choose to imagine that the release of serotonin-related, hallucinogenic chemicals (by the pineal gland) during sleep, served as a neurochemical 'kick' that recalls the memory of the drug experience, the chemical effect of which was similar to dreaming. Whatever way we approach our analysis there is certainly room for further research. This is especially true of the link between psychedelic experience, serotonin and sleep.

MDMA has many other less well known but fascinating effects. Ecstasy acts as a short term hay-fever (and indeed general anti-inflammatory) cure. This phenomena has been observed by me with many other users. Indeed the general pain-killing effects of MDMA are well established. Again we should examine the effect in both psychological *and* physiological terms (neurochemically there is a link between histamine production, that is related to allergic reactions, and the serotonin system which MDMA effects). The pain killing effect of MDMA (which happens without the sort of somatic disassociation associated with many other pain-killers), as well as the tendency for many users to revel in rhythm, could mean that MDMA (or a variation of this chemical) may have use as a drug for mothers in labour. (Animal experiments have shown no significant findings - in terms of evident damage to off-spring - where MDMA was fed to pregnant laboratory rats). In human terms some female users report that Ecstasy can bring on their period and that it can (on occasion) lead to periods which are heavier than normal.[233] Ecstasy has certainly already been useful in helping people with terminal illness remain alert, calm, and free of pain without the need for disassociating morphine treatment.

As LSD breaks apart reality so MDMA blurs its edges. This blurring of boundaries does not mean that we are 'shaken up' with the boundary destroying power of a major psychedelic. Instead strangers begin to look familiar (mistaken identity is common in clubs!), the lights blur and the dissolution of being on the dance floor or sitting chilling out is felt to be a series of movements in a symphony of activity rather than isolated vignettes of time. The blurring of boundaries that MDMA facilitates can been seen in club art and style, where fluorescent light and costume serve to stimulate clubbers by aping the effect of the drug itself.

The empathic quality of MDMA makes it the perfect drug for verbally processing ideas, especially ideas where the emotional content would normally swamp the very act of communicating. For this reason psychotherapy, counselling and divination are ideal uses of this drug. Writing (or at least the formation of ideas into linear narratives) also flows well when on ecstasy, especially towards the end of the trip when the 'speedy' effects are generally reduced and the mind is somewhat quieter.

In a magical sense MDMA can allow us to formulate ideas clearly and then let them go. These may be 'spells' cast into the unconscious mind (or 'self affirmations' it you prefer a more psychological description).

# Amphetamine

'Speed is the poor man's' cocaine' commented a friend of mine. This is certainly the way that speed is usually perceived in western culture. As a central nervous system stimulant speed provides a 'buzz', a 'kick' and, if the circumstances are right, a 'rush'.

The amphetamine class of chemicals covers a broad church, from methylphenidate (trade name Ritalin) through to the crystallised form of methylamphetamine (known as 'Ice' or 'Euphoria'). Depending on the set, setting and substance variables, speed can have a range of effects. The most common are a general 'pepping up', without necessarily any feeling of having changed or challenged ones usual sense of being. However it would be a mistake to imagine that speed does not contain its own transcendent power. My own experience of Ice in particular (taken orally in solution) is that there is a psychedelic-type component to the speed experience. This can include a sense not simply of confidence and alertness, but a direct feeling that one is, in every way engaged with the world. Unlike the dreamy quality of many hallucinogenic experiences, speed brings everything into focus, into sharp and sometimes stark relief.

The physical and psychological range of effects that speed can generate is well known. From 'shrivelling up' the penis in men, the 'speed shakes', the strange electrical feeling in the roots of one's hair as though one's scalp has become electrically charged, and of course talking, talking, talking...

Speed, like cocaine, has tremendous uses as an appetite suppressant and general stimulant. It can be combined effectively with a number of other drugs, the most common being its use to heighten the energetic side of MDMA's effect. Ice has been recommended by some writers: '...it is said to help concentration and thinking - a sort of "make-you-smarter" drug, with a minor speed-like component to it.'[234] For some users, notably those who favour injecting as their preferred route of administration, the rush is the attraction. Rather than a fairly gentle stimulant (which speed can be, depending on dose and particularly when taken orally) it is the hard and fast sense of 'powering up' that the intravenous speed user seeks out.

Tolerance to speed develops fairly quickly in most people. The after effects of speed, particularly if it has been consumed as part of a 'run' (perhaps three days of continuous partying or working) can be fairly nasty. Aggressive feelings can be released by speed. For many people this seems to be doubly so if amphetamine use is combined with alcohol. The aggressive 'gnarly' feeling that amphetamine can provoke might be generated as part of the come down (the user senses their 'loss' of this heightened engagement with the world and mourns this). It may also be due to physical fatigue and tiredness.

The 'fiery' side of speed may be due to its chemical effect on the central nervous system and on norepinephrine.[235] This acts on the hypothetical basic instincts of the 'flight, fright, flight, fuck' responses. Again, depending on circumstances, amphetamine can have the effect of stimulating sexual desire (though often impeding the ability to orgasm) or it may directly inhibit erection in men. In women speed, particularly its stronger forms (such as Ice), can disrupt the menstrual cycle. In some cases a powerful amphetamine experience will stop a period dead in its tracks. This may lead to the following period being heavier or more likely to be accompanied by menstrual cramp.

The speed high (especially if the high is a powerful one from smoked or injected forms of amphetamine) can be very addictive. Yet it is the sense of control, of self-possession that is perhaps the most difficult thing for the speed addict to give up. Used intelligently, amphetamines can clear, focus and sustain the mind. Used inappropriately it can serve as an object lesson in the law of diminishing returns.

## Cocaine

'If something is worth its weight in gold then that's not really that valuable. But if it's worth its weight in coke then it really is expensive!' As this remark exemplifies, one of the fundamental parts of the cocaine experience is the cost. The sense of decadence and richness which surrounds the purchase and use of cocaine is paralleled by the euphoric and subtly enchanting effect of the drug. And what is it that cocaine makes you want to do? 'Cocaine makes you want to take more cocaine!'

Coming from a relatively small part of the globe (*Erythroxylon coca* grows between 1,500 and 6,000 feet above sea level in cool, humid, frost-free conditions with little annual temperature variation) cocaine is (globally speaking) a rare and sought after material. Its use (in the form of chewed leaves) dates back many thousands of years. In the mountainous regions that the drug hails from it is ideal to help native people endure fatigue (caused by lack of oxygen at these altitudes) and the chill winds. In its green leaf form coca contains a rich complex of vitamins and trace minerals (leading more than one friend to comment that 'cocaine: it's not a drug, it's the perfect food!'). Sadly the high intensity (and, of course, illegal) production of cocaine means that the crop is currently responsible for farming practices which cause large scale environmental damage.[236]

It is possible to take cocaine, like most drugs, in a variety of ways. But by far the most common today is by 'snorting'. Because of the expense of cocaine street 'end user' supplies are often heavily adulterated. The main reason for this is to bulk the product out but it may also be done in order to introduce other drugs into the mixture that give the appearance of the coke being 'good stuff'. The reason for this is that the cocaine hit is subtle in the extreme. Freud, when he wrote about cocaine, (he was taking his orally in solution) called it a 'magical drug', declaring that:

> Long-lasting, intensive mental or physical work can be performed without fatigue…it is as though the need for food and sleep, which otherwise makes itself felt peremptorily at certain times of the day, were completely banished…The psychic effect consists of exhilaration and lasting euphoria, which does not differ in any way from the normal euphoria of a healthy person…one senses an increase in self-control and feels more vigorous and more capable of work…one is simply normal, and soon finds it difficult to believe that one is under the influence of any drug at all.[237]

This is the central point about cocaine. It is a drug that creates a 'normal' state of mind. Even the initial rush of snorting or injecting is short lived. Chemically cocaine stimulates the peripheral nervous system (and probably the central nervous system). It also acts upon dopamine and norepinephrine. Depending on dose its physical effects can include a rise in body temperature, vasoconstruction and accelerated heartbeat. At higher doses (and with the right set and setting) cocaine can have subtle hallucinogenic effects. The world seems clearer, the Self more connected and in-control. Colours may appear brighter but there is no sense that the phenomena is 'external' in the way that these changes would be construed with LSD or mushrooms. The world does not become 'weird', but 'hyper-authentic' – and you're in control. The first time that I took a decent sized line I felt myself somehow 'taller', a sensation that was powerful in itself but lacked the complexities of meaning that I would have attached to it were it to have happened with a conventional psychedelic.

Coke can be psychologically addictive but this addiction must be learnt. One must develop a taste for cocaine in order to get the most out of it. Robert Sabbag expresses the subtlety and learnt attraction of cocaine by pointing out that:

> Cocaine has no edge. It is strictly a motor drug. It does not alter your perception; it will not even wire you up like the amphetamines. No pictures, no time/space warping, no danger, no fun, no edge…Coke is to acid what jazz is to rock. You have to appreciate it. *It* does not come to *you*.[238]

Most users, once they acquire 'the taste' are keenly aware of how 'things go better with coke' and that the insidious attraction (which is both the bane and beauty of coke) must be monitored so that it does not get out of hand. For most people the pragmatic necessity of eating and paying bills means that coke is simply too expensive to develop a serious habit. Of course we are all aware of how this can change when a position of financial superiority is reached (whether it be financed by work in the concert hall or the City).

As already mentioned cocaine is a notorious aphrodisiac, though some men experience a paradoxical effect (short term impotence) with its use. For women the sexual effect of cocaine is usually that it promotes confidence and is an 'aid' to sexual arousal. Some women experience vaginal dryness with cocaine, an effect that can also happen with large doses of caffeine or amphetamine.

The smokable 'free base' form of cocaine is of course crack. Whilst crack has become in recent years the new 'devil drug' of the British media its effects are pretty much the same as those of snorted cocaine. The only difference is the speed and height of the initial rush. The effects of crack are more pronounced than snorted coke but wear off sooner. As with any stimulant high many users find that the greater the rush, the higher the peak, the more rapid and unpleasant the come down.

Excessive use of cocaine (in whatever form) can lead to paranoia and 'psychotic' states of mind, but again this outcome is not simply caused by the drug but must be supported by the contribution of set and setting. For instance, with crack it is primarily the combination of the short and high rush, coupled with the social circumstances of users in a 'culture of desperation', that can lead to violent situations. Crack itself is no more a 'bad' drug than alcohol, hashish or LSD.

Cocaine is certainly a useful, enjoyable drug and, once one acquires a taste for it, can be treated like good quality wine. Its effect in clearing the mind and focusing concentration is unparalleled.

One effect of cocaine's 'ego centred' high is that it can reduce the effect of psychedelic drugs. In the case of LSD I find that even a fairly small amount of coke will significantly reduce the effect of acid. Although I've never tried coke as an 'antidote' to a hallucinogenic it may well be effective in this respect. When coke is used with MDMA it tends to enhance the 'dopamine' or 'Self' focused effects of ecstasy. The 'loved up' fluffy empathogenic quality of the MDMA is reduced, whereas the drive to dance and the general stimulant effect is enhanced.

Of course the joys of cocaine are not for everyone. A good friend remarked that snorting cocaine, 'produced a clearing of the mind' but he felt a, 'dislike of any drug whose initial effects are like the first symptoms of a head cold!'

# Opium
> There may seem to be some contradiction in the use of drugs and a belief in yoga and meditation. There is. Life is full of contraction.

> Yet the drugs/yoga contradiction seems less hypocritical and less injurious, less misleading than the wealth/yoga and power/yoga contradictions illustrated by professional holy men and other religious leaders...I always fixed with my left hand. Drugs belong to the left-handed path, the path of Shakti.[239] The junk seemed to hit me right between the eyes...That was my special spot, the seat of the intuition, of the higher facilities of mind. Mind, mentation, misery, madness, Maya. This was my scene. I am trapped in mind...Next I could smell the junk inside my nose, then feel it in my throat, constricting it, causing me to swallow hard...and finally there was a twitch of the rectum as it readjusted to the new biochemical status quo of my body. Then the snake rose again, and instantly it was at the top of the trail, exploding like a soothing star-cluster in the skull, healing nectar pouring down into every nerve of the network.

This account of the use of speed and smack in the context of 'left hand path' yoga, by Jasper Newsome, is not atypical of opiate drug stories.[240] However much the British government's campaign in the 1980s served to remove the glamour of heroin, its transgressive power has resurfaced again and again. Whether it be the continuing revival in the magically inspired works of William Burroughs or currently of Will Self, within the film *Trainspotting*, or the heroin chic of the cat walk.

From its first mention in ancient Sumeria, the opium poppy and its pharmaceutical derivatives have had a strange and, at times strained, relationship with humanity. There can be no doubt that the figure of the addict, especially the intravenous using junkie, is a powerful spectre in western culture. Yet the demon drug itself, morphine, is one of the most commonly employed (though by no means one hundred percent effective) painkiller in medical use.[241]

In its addictive use opiates 'promise nothing'. Heroin allows the user to return to the womb, to a place in which nothing matters; not hunger, not poverty, not pain, not others.

The opiates are not without their own brand of psychedelic effects, and can produce all manner of 'visionary' experiences. The possibility of hallucinatory effects seem most pronounced with opium in its 'raw' form (especially if eaten rather than smoked). In general the visions offer a sombre and awful sense of scale and grandeur. Opium visions are not the communal psychedelia of an acid house party or of ecstasy fuelled rave. 'Solitude and silence', as De Quincey[242] puts it, are the ideal conditions in which to experience it. The opium poppy is quintessentially a drug of the night, of the chthonic spaces described in the novels of H.P.Lovecraft. Unlike the wheeling musings of cannabis, or lightning quick, multi-dimensional thoughts of LSD, opium allows the user to pursue an idea until it is annihilated into a Zen-like nothingness.

Opiates work chemically by mimicking the pain killing chemicals present in the body. They also seem to affect the so-called 'pain-pleasure' systems in the brain. Currently research is focused around the effect of opiates on dopamine which some neurochemists have described as 'the substance that helps convert the neurochemical spells of drugs into the brain's own language and pleasure.'[243] In terms of the functional duality of serotonin (Other)/dopamine (Self) one could hypothesise that dopamine, as the focus (by the mind) for the processes of Self, is the chemical that means we ('I') can become happy or sad depending on the presence of a stimulus (e.g. food, sex, cold, death etc.). After all one cannot have a sense of pleasure unless there is a sense of 'I' (however 'fictional' it may be in absolutist or cognitive terms) to 'have' that sense. Although the rush and glow of the heroin trip can dissolve ones sense of Self (and potentially lead to unconsciousness) the experience of heroin, as a whole, is of a drug that defends the boundaries of Self. (Indeed the word 'heroin' is derived from 'heroic' which is how the first people it was tested on consistently reported they felt.) Unlike LSD or MDMA, opiates do not 'shake up' ones sense of Self, rather they cocoon it, perhaps to the point of sleep. In any case the boundary between Self and Other is reaffirmed by the drug experience. Unlike cocaine where the boundary between Self and Other is populated by feelings of frenetic engagement and sense of potency, opiates work by creating a void, an *absence* of importance or meaning between Self and Other. For this reason opiates can be an amazing way to study the Self isolated and alone. They provide an opportunity to cut ourselves off from the world and examine who we are. Heroin is the drug of the hermit and retreating from the world in this way can certainly lead to powerful insights.

Of course, given the appropriate conditions, the hermitage can easily become a prison. The pain killing effect of opiates mean that they are powerful addictive drugs. They inculcate themselves so well with the body so that it is famously known that - assuming you had an inexhaustible supply of good smack, a reliable method of ingesting it and someone to remind you to eat on hand - heroin causes few if any deleterious effects on the body. This is why heroin can be so difficult to give up, aside of the psychological addiction (and I'll let the distinction stand unchallenged for the purposes of the argument) heroin fits like the perfect key in the chemistry of the body. Opiates serve to mimic and, in time, reduce the production of, endorphins in the mid-brain areas.[244] Indeed new research suggests that actual opiate chemicals may be endogenously present in the body. Perhaps the only other drug that may occur endogenously is DMT which, in contrast to opium, produces little or no subjective tolerance (especially when smoked) and no withdrawal. DMT may well be to the serotonin system as opium is to dopamine.

The fact that significant opium use reduces the body's own pain relieving chemicals makes it perfectly intelligible why withdrawal from opiate addiction is so physically painful. In one respect one might use the psychoanalytical model that much of what a new-born individual experiences, and learns to reduce (by a series of strategies) is anxiety. Anxiety is 'the pain of impotence' and, in the case of psychosomatic illnesses, can be directly translated by the mind into physical pain. If the desire to reduce anxiety by behaviours (both observable outward and internal strategies) is essential to the development of an individuated Self then a drug that reduces anxiety chemically (opium) is likely to be very attractive. Moreover if we think of sensation itself (including physical sensation) as being a form of 'pain' (i.e. being subject to the psychic processes of anxiety and repression) then total reduction of anxiety means reduction of all pain, and therefore of all feeling (whether positive/desired or negative/feared). The very physical sensations which we learn to cope with and even enjoy are deadened by opium; it effectively kills emotional turmoil as well as it dulls physical distress. The reduction in anxiety means the removal of the very basis of feeling, namely the knowledge of the uncontrollable Other (in Freudian terms 'the breast' that 'goes away'). Opiates may lead towards a form of pleasure, but this pleasure is distinctly one of *lack*. The pleasure is that of release, of nothing, of the Self made unrelated to the world and contained once more in the womb of pre-anxiety, existence. This is the most fun you can have from unconsciousness without (necessarily being) unconscious. If we take Freud's view, that the primary anxiety is that of the birth experience, then again we see how the idea of morphine as taking the user 'back to the womb' fits in well with this description.

Once the mind and body learns that it can locate its way of dealing with anxiety so exactly within the exogenous (i.e. outside the body) opiate it ceases to be able to generate the pain-killing response in itself. Thus the 'physical addiction' to opium is born.

Psychologically the process of learning to depend on opiates is amazingly enhanced by the use of a hypodermic needle to administer the drug. Indeed the complex of ideas surrounding intravenous use of opium are legion. Although the quality and speed of the initial rush are enhanced by this method of delivery, it is perhaps the powerful nexus of discourse centred around the act of injecting drugs that is more significant. Discourses about vampirism, the death drive, the autopoiesis of the body (using the tool of medicine to create a self inscribed 'writing on the body'), the transgression of social tabu, and more are grouped together in the symbolic act of 'shooting up'. It is often said by drugs workers, and rightly so, that the needle is as addictive as the drug. Of course many other drugs can and are injected, with cocaine and speed being perhaps the most commonly employed. But neither drug, in cultural terms, represents so much of a statement about human mortality as shooting smack. To become truly oneself, free from anxiety, suspended over the pit of death, of Morpheus, is the project of the intravenous user. Mainlining exemplifies the pleasure and pain of drug use perhaps more powerfully than any other drug in our culture. No matter how unglamorous the life of the poverty stricken addict, the glamour of opium is undoubtedly still going strong today.

## Ketamine

Ketamine is 'used mainly for anaesthesia in children, but it is also used for induction of anaesthesia and its analgesic properties are of value in the management of patients with severe burns requiring skin grafts. Vivid dreams and hallucinations may occur during the recovery period.'[245] Or, to put the point differently, as a close friend remarked, 'before I took

Ketamine I wondered why people took pre-med. for fun. Now I wonder why they give Ketamine to people in hospitals! Ketamine is a disassociative hypnotic and anaesthetic. At low doses or during the recovery from a higher knock-out dose, ketamine can set the sense of self free from the physical structure of the body.

The effects of ketamine means that the location of the physical body is eroded. The Self (which can appear bodiless or clothed within a morphing, ghostly, imaginative replica of the actual body) may have the sense of flying, falling, spinning or stretching out for miles then becoming tiny, microscopic or atomic.

Ketamine acts rapidly (it is most often taken orally or snorted though some users favour intravenous or intramuscular administration), it is characterised by profound analgesia, mild cardiac stimulation and respiratory depression. Unlike other anaesthetics, protective reflexes such as coughing and swallowing are maintained. This is of great significance since many drug related deaths are caused by excessive use 'of various substances' leading to unconsciousness and suffocation, often as a result of inhaling vomit.

When snorted, the ketamine hit is like being plunged into a psychedelic experience. The colours of the world are subtly turned up a notch and there is a general sense of 'weirdness'. Although it can be taken in a social setting, ketamine is predominately an inward, personal experience. As well as spatial hallucinations and dissociation, ketamine can give rise to visual hallucinations of a distinctly psychedelic type. My own experience of the drug is that the visuals tend to be more austere, saturnine and simplistic, with a Zen-like quality about them. Visuals might include scenes but without the general lushness or colour of LSD closed eye visuals. More common are abstract figures, shapes which tend towards monochromes or muted colours, often with a vaguely mathematical quality about them (as though they were elaborate diagrams or complex geometric mandalas).

The sense of leaving ones body with ketamine may be both the explanation for, and the gateway into, near death experiences. Certainly it may be the case that some patients who have found themselves looking down on their bodies in the operating theatre may have received ketamine as part of their treatment. Again establishing cause and effect is difficult (does ketamine induce these visions or simply mimic them?). The ketamine experience, whilst not necessarily frightening (in fact, although inward, it can be riotously funny) does have the feel of death about it, the sense of 'shuffling off this mortal coil' is profound. It may certainly be of interest to magicians who wish to explore shamanic flight or other forms of 'out of body' experiences.

## Cigarettes & Alcohol
## (...and tea, coffee, chocolate and sugar)

Though use has reached epidemic proportions in the west (and, increasingly, global culture) these drugs can certainly be used for transgressive ritual.

Tobacco has perhaps the best known heritage, having been used by Native American peoples for hundreds of years as a sacred drug. Varieties of tobacco that have a more profound, possibly hallucinogenic effect, have been commented on by some writers.[246] However, even a cigarette from the corner shop can be a tool for magical translation.[247] Smoking behind the bike sheds, and indulging in this most commonplace of addictions, is a right of passage for many young people.

Sugar is generally one of the first (in terms of the individual's history) drug experiences. And, as anyone who does not usually consume much sugar will testify, the 'sugar rush', and subsequent come down, are very real experiences.

The comforting glow of chocolate and the alert state promoted by coffee should also never be undervalued. Indeed, the history of *Theobroma cacao,* (the original 'food of the gods') has been examined by writer Jonathan Ott, who discusses the 'nutritional, pharmacologic and aphrodisiac qualities' of chocolate.[248] Like tobacco, chocolate has a range of effects, and in a society where there is an emphasis not on mass-produced quantity but on quality, relationship and 'refining your rapture', these drugs can certainly have important esoteric and cultural effects.

This complex history of those drugs that are not currently prohibited in western society is certainly worthy of examination. We should not naively assume that the legality of these drugs is due to their (relatively) gentle effects. It is true that none of the above drugs are psychedelic when consumed in moderate doses. But the effect on a user during their first few experiences with these drugs, or of a high dose, can be dramatic. In the periods during which these drugs became established within culture, any significant drug experiences associated with them would have almost certainly have been stronger, since the drug experience was not 'defined' within the established discourses of society. In some sense, because the 'meaning' of coffee (for instance) was not yet established, the high that it produced was apt to be more variable in its form and perhaps, in some cases, stronger. In 1511 during the reign of the European Prince Waldeck, he offered a reward to people who would inform the authorities of illegal coffee drinkers. Even as late as 1777 European authorities were prepared to license the clergy and aristocracy the delight of coffee use but not the lower classes, who might be fined and publicly flogged for its use.[249] These laws would certainly have had a cultural effect on users. In much the same way that modern cocaine users undoubtedly derive part of their pleasure from the decadence and illegality of their snorting. These drugs certainly provided a focus for new social interactions. During the Enlightenment, the coffee house became the meeting place of the chattering classes, and was looked upon with disdain by more conservative members in society.

Tobacco (as part of the cannabis joint) can be employed as the carrier material for the consumption of cannabis. Coffee and chocolate can be used as the materials into which other powerful drugs (such as cannabis oil in coffee, or dope in hash truffles) may be blended. This creates a synergy which enhances the effect of both drugs.

Alcohol, that most ancient of drugs, can also be used as the 'carrier' for other drugs (Champagne with MDMA powder dissolved into it is a particularly poetic example of this practice). The effects of alcohol alone can have wide and often paradoxical variations, the same basic drug producing various effects whether it is consumed as gin, tequila slammers, or supped as a pint of beer. For some people, alcohol provides them with just the same insights and transgressive potentials that are normally accorded only to drugs like LSD. One friend, who is a writer, told me that he finds his 'best poetry and best ideas' come from wine. Alcohol tends to break down and blur boundaries in much the same way as MDMA (accounting for its disinhibiting and emotional effects). Unlike MDMA, in most users, the alternate stimulant and depressant effects of the drug means that the alcohol 'trip' can become unstable. This leads to the swings of emotion commonly associated with drinking, first laughter, then earnestness, perhaps aggression and sometimes depression. As with all drugs, and perhaps especially with alcohol, we are faced with the fact that the set, setting and substance can lead to wide variations in experience.

## 2-CB

Derived from the same set of phenethylamines of which MDMA is a member, 2-CB is another remarkable drug. It is certainly hallucinogenic at the right dose and can give rise to bright and colourful visuals. However, its most remarkable effect is that it is a somatic hallucinogen. Unlike ketamine, the changes in perception it brings are not of the disassociate variety. Instead, most users report an enhanced sense of being in their bodies – physical, tactile, smell and taste sensations are all enhanced. For some users this is the ideal aphrodisiac since it enhances body sensations, and has a generally 'up' or stimulant quality. Unlike MDMA, where erection in men tends to be reduced, and where orgasm for both sexes may be difficult to achieve, 2-CB has no such drawbacks.

A 'fact sheet' on 2-CB[250] details some of its effects:

> ...Another aspect of the 2C-B experience, apparently common to all experimenters, is an intensification of the senses of touch, smell, taste; an increased response to colour and sound. As with many psychoactive materials, there is a degree of anaesthesia which affects the pain-receptors in the skin, particularly. Pinching the inside of the knee, for instance, produces little discomfort, and care must be taken to warn a patient not to touch a heated object which would ordinarily cause him to withdraw his hand reflexively; under 2C-B, especially at higher levels, he might not perceive the heat immediately and a burn could result. Paradoxically, the perception of the faintest touch on the skin is heightened considerably, and physical discomfort or pain resulting from a broken bone or any kind of strain or imbalance in the body tends to be increased. Some people have reported the use of 2C-B as a diagnostic aid or ally, since it enables an increased perception of problems present in the body, when attention is turned in that

direction. There is insufficient data, at present, on this potentially useful aspect of 2C-B, and we hope that more will be available in time.

Perceptions of imbalance - either physical or emotional in kind - tend to take the forms of images often intense, colourful and in some cases, overwhelming. If the therapist is not taking the 2C-B with his patient, he will need well-educated antennae and a reservoir of emotional warmth to help his patient structure and assimilate and understand the experience.

In small doses it is a stimulant and may well act on the 'reptile' (i.e. the limbic system and the 'lower' regions) areas within the brain (or mind…). Small doses of 2-CB provide perhaps the best synergy with MDMA if you want to dance the night away. Although commonly people tend to use amphetamine to prolong and provide the stimulant component of a night's 'raving', speed can easily dull the psychedelic edge of MDMA and can produce a physically and psychologically difficult come down. 2-CB as an alternative can help to provide the 'animal energy' needed for clubbing, but without reducing the empathogenic, entactogenic or psychedelic aspects of Ecstasy.

In larger doses the effect on the primal reptile brain can mean an activation of what might be thought of as our basic drives. This experience can be very disturbing. Generally doses of 25mg are thought of as a general rule-of-thumb upper limit. Doses in excess of some 45mg are know to produce difficult to handle effects. The main problem with large doses of 2-CB is that there is a generalised feeling of terror or fear. This may be due to the hallucinogenic action of the drug stimulating the reptile brain. It may be possible to creatively channel this evocation of ones 'basic drives' into physical exercise or feats of endurance, fighting or sex.[251]

## Ibogaine

Ibogaine is obtained from two related tree genera in South America and Africa. It is in West Africa that the drug's use has the longest history. Outside of the more occult drug circles and the pharmaceutical and medical professions, ibogaine is little known. At least for the moment.

The Multidisciplinary Association for Psychedelic Studies (MAPS) archive on the internet describes ibogaine's effects in three parts: 'The first is a four to six hour period emulating dreaming, in which either visual presentations or thoughts dealing with past events are experienced. The second is a cognitive or intellectual period in which those experiences are evaluated and the third is a period of residual stimulation eventually resulting in sleep. It is after the patient awakes that the effects are principally noticed, with a lack of a desire in the majority of patients, to seek or use the drugs they were abusing.'

It is this last point that is so important. Consistently, clinical trials have shown that ibogaine can change addictive patterns of behaviour.[252] Evidence for this comes from both human and animal studies. Ibogaine appears to be able to 'cure' addiction. Its power seems to work across the board, with studies showing that ibogaine can alleviate both the physiological and psychological effects of addiction. Material at MAPS addresses this paradoxical ability. 'What they [cocaine and opiates] do share in common…is that use of either substance increases dopaminergic (DA) activity in the brain's mesolimbic system, and/or mesocortical pathways. This triggers the reward mechanism, which is associated with the reinforcing effects of drugs of abuse. Researchers thus began looking at the relationship of ibogaine to the DA system. To date, studies have examined cocaine, opiate, nicotine and alcohol addictions and found that ibogaine is effective in treating all these. Researchers have found that "ibogaine significantly decreased the intensity of many withdrawal signs" in rats addicted to morphine.'[253]

Although, as writer Andrew Tyler points out, 'The touting of one drug as cure for dependence on another is a recurring theme in pharmacological history,'[254] it may well be that ibogaine represents an important candidate for treating drug addiction. Indeed some researchers have gone beyond the notion of drug addiction and suggest that ibogaine may represent a treatment for *addiction itself*.[255] Obviously this would mean that we have on our hands a psychoactive drug that would threaten the very basis of global capitalist culture. It remains to be seen how the transgressive and economic history of this material will unfold.

The ibogaine trip begins from doses of 200-300mg. Some individuals take a single dose of 700-1800mg resulting in a 24-38hr psychoactive period. In native use, the Fang of West Africa typically use one large dose as an initiatory ritual to 'open the head'. Thereafter lower doses are used. Larger doses seem to have the greatest effect, in terms of the inner psychedelic experience (its depth and duration). In terms of anti-addictive properties it may well be most effective if used as part of anti-addictive therapies. Physically, the ibogaine trance can include dizziness, poor co-ordination, nausea, and vomiting for a short part of the trip for some users. Most users find themselves in a state of drowsiness in which they do not want to move, open their eyes, or attend to the environment. The fascination seems to be the inner dialogue. Again a paper at MAPS quoting pharmacological studies talks of:

> ...an enhancement of fantasy without experiencing changes in the perception of the environment, delusions, depersonalisation, or formal alterations of thinking. Ibogaine's fantasies (often described as a 'movie run at high speed' or 'slide show') were reported as rich in archetypal contents, involving animals and/or the subject

himself with or without other individuals. The fantasies evoked by ibogaine were easy to manipulate by both the subjects and the psychotherapist'

In this way the ibogaine vision could be said to be remarkably similar to a lucid dream. The MAPS writer goes on to say: 'The patients were able to respond to the questions of the therapists. It was concluded that ibogaine could act as a psychological catalyst which could compress a long psychotherapeutic process into a shorter time.'[256].

Again, studies on rats do not reveal how important this internal dialogue may be as part of the anti-addictive process of ibogaine. This may be another example of the drug paradox; that it is the psychic effect of the drug that 're-tuned' the reward pathways in the brain, as much as it is a 'bottom up' chemical effect on behaviour. Moreover, as with ketamine, the effect of the inner psychedelic experience of ibogaine is going to be difficult to establish if your subject is a rat.[257]

# Wild Wood

At the borders of usual drug experimentation there is a huge range of drugs, many of which require specialist knowledge or home cultivation, that may be explored. There is, for example, a large number of psychedelic cacti (many of which can be discreetly purchased in both Europe and the USA). There are number of mushrooms besides the usual 'liberty cap' which are psychoactive, including fly agaric. Equally, acid-like experiences are to be had from the morning glory plant, visions from the humble decorative plant *pipiltzintzintli* (or 'coleus') and of course the powerful solanaceous plants (such as the daturas). There are stimulants too, such as the plant *khat (Celastrus edulis)*.

Although 'natural' the user should never mistake the power of organic drugs as being inherently any different from 'artificial' chemicals (look at how powerful raw opium is compared to the very mild consciousness changes usually associated with synthetic paracetamol). Although dosage is more problematic with a plant than with a purified chemical, a prudent approach and good reading around the proposed drug for experimentation does reduce the dangers of unpleasant effects.[258]

There are significant advantages to growing or gathering your own drugs. One is that you can consciously develop a rich and complex relationship with the plant. The relationship is not only with the drug and drug experience, but the broader experiences of gathering, farming, harvesting and identification of the plant also.

In pragmatic terms, home production also means not paying money to disreputable criminal cartels, indirectly supporting governmental and other groups for whom drugs are just another product. Trying to reduce the amount of time and energy that one expends supporting these power-structures and unsustainable farming practices is energy well spent. But this does not necessarily mean that someone who smokes home produced weed and uses local mushrooms is inherently a better human being.

Some drugs would be difficult to produce in any other way than by complex pharmaceutical methods (such as MDMA). In these cases I am personally perfectly happy to buy these from a distant supplier. However, as with any other product, it would be good to know that the supplier was: a) manufacturing and trading ethically and in as sustainable a way as possible b) that, in a taxed economy, due taxation is raised from the sale of the product and used in appropriate social investment.

People who use drugs, I feel, must recognise the need to legalise them, but they should be aware that this is a global trade (no different from the trade in computer chips or cotton) and not just think of the problem in terms of 'end-user' use. As with any trade moral and political considerations should apply.

## Mindgames

The use of drugs can of course include polydrug use and there is a certain art of the blending together of different chemicals to produce different states. The production of different forms of alcoholic beverage, and different combinations of chocolate and coffee alone demonstrate this.

Certain drugs have a powerful synergy together – such as MDMA and LSD or amphetamine and alcohol. In exploring the transgressive potential of drugs the magician must beware certain combinations of drugs that can have dangerous or even fatal consequences. MAO inhibitors can potentiate the effect of some drugs but can cause fatal hypertensive crisis. Whilst some combinations such as cocaine and valium end up pulling the mind and body of the drug taker in two different directions at once; with the dramatic consequences witnessed by the death of actor River Phoenix.

When using drugs, one must be conscious of the broad definition of drugs, which includes many substances that we usually think of as foods. For example powerful MAO inhibitors are to be found in sauerkraut, whereas the laxative effect of chewing gum can exacerbate the tendency of some people on MDMA to have loose bowel movements.

When taking any drug it is advisable to keep consumption of other foods and chemicals under scrutiny. This may be part of the reason that, in many cultures, abstinence from anything other than a very simple diet (and often fasting) is recommended before a sacred drug is taken.

Polydrug use can be a useful experience. In the case of alcohol and amphetamine synergy one can experience being drunk, followed by moments of speed-high activity and lucidity, and then back into alcoholic fuzz. By combining different drugs one can see their differences clearly as well as the points at which they (and therefore the structures within the mind of the drug taker) coincide.

# The Modern Things:
# drugs, transgression and society

### Babylon's Burning

A detailed discussion of the politics of drug use is outside the scope of this book. However, the place of drugs within the political economy of society, should not be dismissed as unimportant to the individual pursuing a magical engagement with drugs. If drugs are to be our helpers, our allies and our teachers then we should not trade them with the contempt usually reserved by colonials for dealing in slaves.

Writer Brian Inglis sums up the position of many people who are either users of, or concerned about, the current illegal drugs trade.

> Endlessly over the last past few years, the issue has been debated; should cannabis, or mescaline, or LSD be legalised? The record of history suggests that the question should be put the other way round; should such drugs be banned? For then, the answer can be given unequivocally: no. Prohibition has always failed in free enterprise societies – free, that is, to the extent that consumers who have the means can exercise freedom of choice. If they choose drugs, no law can stop them. Prohibition may restrict supplies, for a time, but that will only drive prices up, bringing in

> fresh supplies – or different drugs. And this flouting of the law breeds disrespect for it, alienates otherwise law-abiding citizens, and corrupts the law enforcers...
>
> Drug use, and drug abuse, are a reflection of society, its tensions, its values, and its needs. To punish drug-takers is like a drunk striking the bleary face which he sees in the mirror. Drugs will not be brought under control until society itself changes, enabling men to use them as primitive man did; welcoming the visions they provided not as fantasies, but as intimations of a different, and important, level of reality. It is not reached by drugs alone; techniques such as meditation may provide a more satisfying approach. But at least, taken for this purpose, they can give the initial illumination; the first introduction to unexplored reaches of the mind.[259]

'The Drug Problem' that many people seem (out of fear and ignorance) to want to deal with by a 'War on Drugs', serves to obscure the real issues of addiction, social deprivation, illegal trade systems and to ignore the desire for transgression as fundamentally part of the human spirit. The moral drive to legalise drugs does come, in some quarters, from a libertarian attitude. Simply; 'I've got a right to take drugs and it's none of the State's concern'. However the State *is* and *should* be concerned with human problems, especially the grief that can arise from drug addiction. It is precisely for this reason that we should legalise all drugs, so that we can take conscious control and responsibility for this trade and not keep sticking our heads in the sand.

In the context of a libertarian basis for drug law reform, Leary proposes his '5th freedom' ('to change one's consciousness'). The aim being, to extend the existing four fundamental freedoms proposed by F.D.Roosevelt ('freedom of speech and expression, freedom of worship, freedom from want, freedom from fear'). This is all well and good but we must ask ourselves, in the pragmatic context of supply and demand, at what cost these freedoms and in what way can we realise them? In order not to compromise one individual's freedom at the expense of another, we must ask how that freedom is most readily and morally gained. In asking for the fifth freedom we must acknowledge the pragmatic responsibilities that that entails. Social responsibilities to inform others and to act with discretion and honour in our use of drugs. And economic responsibilities to ensure that what we are sniffing, smoking and injecting isn't making one person rich and another person poor and destroying the ecology of the earth in its production.[260]

Certainly the use of drugs can be dangerous, but never more so than in societies where the human drive to transgress and engage with the sacred, the 'Real' is socially thwarted. The human project to transgress, to explore the self will lead to blind excess if it fails to be culturally supported. A good example of this danger is identified by Matthew Collin (with John Godfrey) in their excellent history of the 'rave scene':

> On the Scottish hardcore scene, stories abounded of young ravers mixing prescription sedatives like Temazepam with Buckfast tonic wine, 'E' and speed. As the music got faster, the exertion more frenzied and strenuous, it was perhaps no coincidence that the hardcore honeymoon period of 1991 saw the highest yet number of Ecstasy-related deaths, just as the first Ecstasy fatalities in Holland followed the development of the hyperspeed Lowlands hardcore known as gabber a few years later.[261]

Writer Simon Reynolds goes on to comment on the socio-economic politics of the 'ghost dance' of early 90s rave 'Ardkore culture:

> Amidst the socio-economic deterioration of a Britain well into its second decade of one-party rule, where alternatives seem unimaginable, horizons grow ever narrower, and there's no constructive outlet for anger, what is there left but to zone out, to go with the flow, to *disappear*? There's also an inchoate fury in the

music that comes out in an urge for total release from constraints, a lust for explosive exhilaration. 'Ardkore frenzy is where the somnambulist youth of Britain snap out of the living death of the nineties to grasp at a few moments of fugitive bliss. 'Ardkore seethes with a RAGE TO LIVE, to cram all the intensity absent from a week of drudgery into a few hours of fervour. It's a quest to reach escape velocity.[262]

A sane society is not one that does not use drugs, rather it is one in which drug use is acknowledged, supported and cared for. Moreover, it would be a society in which the transgressive, the magical is recognised and appreciated. For when this is not done the 'fuel' of sexuality, of drugs, of transgression is transformed from the flame of insight, into the purely destructive fire of self-immolation.

## Common People

Who are these magicians, these 'psychonauts', who are changing their awareness, who are transgressing with drugs and what relationship do they have to humanity at large.

Magic is both a personal journey of exploration (which may or may not be thought of as having a 'development' or 'progression' within it) and a study that can, and in some respects must, be conducted within culture. This paradox follows with most mystical endeavours, it is only through a personal moment or process of revelation that knowledge of God arises, but that has never stopped religious communities setting up or holy people interacting with the rest of society.

In some respects the magician is in all of us, since the desire to transgress and explore is a fundamental part of what it means to be a human being. This neatly undermines the elitism which is sadly common place in the writings of many 'drug gurus', Huxley, for instance, wanted a low-key approach to the use of drugs for self-exploration, to enable the 'brightest and the best' to enjoy the spiritual revelations of psychedelics. Leary (at least at first) favoured a more direct approach, with psychedelic enlightenment as an absolute right for all. As Matthew Collin recounts:

> It was Leary's methodology that prevailed, with the results that Huxley feared; LSD became a common street drug, used not for intellectual contemplation or scientific study but for pure kicks, and within a few years it was criminalised and academic researchers were barred from investigating its potential.[263]

Leary married his wife Barbara shortly after taking MDMA in 1978. By the dawn of the 80s Leary was talking in the same terms as Huxley about this new drug experience;

> Let's face it, we're talking about an élitist experience...XTC is a drug that is known, by word of mouth, by sophisticated people who sincerely want to attain a high level of self-understanding and empathy. We're talking about dedicated searchers who are entitled, who've earned a bit of XTC. This is why the general public hasn't heard of it. No one wants a sixties situation to develop where sleazy characters hang around college dorms peddling pills they falsely call XTC to lazy thrill-seekers.

Leary says much the same in *Chic* 7/85. Curiously, this public statement is self-defeating, if these individuals really thought (or felt able) to contain themselves in a sort of psychedelic quietism they would surely not have written and lectured as conspicuously as they did. In this way perhaps the drug experience was even stronger then they consciously realised, seeping out into words and history.

Of course it might be objected that in this book, by setting up notions of 'sacred', 'transgressive' or 'magical' drug taking, I am taking part in just the same exclusivism. However, although I am expressing my ideas in a certain way, there are many, many people who are using drugs in just the way I have described, to explore who they are, without needing to know about the existence of any of these 'academic' concepts. The idea that drug experience is sacred is not the same as saying that it needs to be stored up, away from the eyes of the profane. This type of retentive obsession is fundamental in patriarchal thought (be it 'good karma', semen or capital that we are supposed to conserve lest it be wasted upon the earthly world of the profane) but it is not some kind of universal truth. Leary may not have been right that our culture just needed to take psychedelics and 'drop out' but neither is it fair to suggest that the knowledge of these sacred techniques should be owned by a self-perpetuating elite. Even if there were to be such an elite, the problem as ever is simple; *who watches the watchmen?*

Drug exploration is a *communication*. It means opening oneself up to the Other, it means the death of ones old sense of 'I' and the consecration of a new sense of Self. Like the acquisition of language, drug experience is something that we do alone, but like language it is meaningless unless there is a listener.

Drugs are sacred because of their liminality, their power, they are not sacred because their use and knowledge is rare and reserved for an elite. They are sacred precisely because they are commonplace and because we can all engage with them. It's what we take away from that experience; the gold of transmutation of the self, or the lead of bleary eyes and groaning stomach. For most people both sorts of alchemy will occur.

No-one has the right to dictate who should and who should not experiment with their own mind.

## The Drugs Don't Work

Drug experience can be used as easily to harm as it can to heal, to oppress as easily as to enlighten. Drugs in themselves do not call for deification or demonising.

When we make the 'shamanic return' we place our own drug experiences within the culture and society of our time and place. If the drug experience is a powerful one it can be of such force that it disrupts the 'symbolic realm' (in structuralist terms; the cultural field of meaning that we operate in on a daily basis). In these instances the symbolic realm – how we think of things – may require a radical re-write, but we should always be aware that the drug experience itself is not the answer. If it were, then the early claims of Leary would have been right. All we would need to do would be to use LSD to transform the nastiest individual into a Buddha. Drug experience can be profoundly valuable, but it is not the answer to life, the universe and everything. Huxley sums up the role of drug experience well, though in a characteristically careful (one might say, elitist) manner:

> I am not so foolish as to equate what happens under the influence of mescaline or of any other drug, prepared or in the future preparable, with the realisation of the end and ultimate purpose of human life; Enlightenment, the Beatific Vision. All I am suggesting is that the mescaline experience is what the Catholic theologians call 'a gratuitous grace', not necessary to salvation but potentially helpful and to be accepted thankfully, if made available. To be shaken out of the ruts of ordinary perception, to be shown for a few timeless hours the outer and the inner world, not as they appear to an animal obsessed with survival or to a human being obsessed with words and notions, but as they are apprehended, directly and unconditionally, by Mind at Large – this is an experience of inestimable value to everyone and especially to the intellectual.[264]

Many of the claims made for the value of drug experience are closely interwoven with ideas of the day, and this is not surprising. This is especially the case in which advocates of drug experience are trying to normalise what a given drug will do in terms of existing social concerns. For instance, during the early days of LSD it was hailed as a form of aphrodisiac, with college kids being lured in to all manner of orgiastic, polysexual practices by its effect. But Leary is at pains to point out that LSD can be used to 'cure' homosexuality, and , it would seem, also for celibacy, getting people back on track with 'normal' heterosexuality.[265] Richard Alpert (a.k.a. Ram Dass) makes similar claims in *LSD and Sexuality:*

> ...The subject is a person who contacted me by letter and said, 'I am a primarily overt acting homo-sexual and I don't want to be anymore. I've heard about LSD and I think it could help me. Would you work with me?' [after LSD psychotherapy) One year later our subject is now living with a woman...They have been having intercourse every night, except during her periods. He has had two homosexual experiences since that time [of the therapy] and he did them, he said, mostly to test and find out 'where he was at' and whether or not the changes were real. Now he finds he can still involve himself in homosexual experiences but he keeps returning to the heterosexual one and finds it indeed far more satisfying. This is a major change in his perceptual, cognitive, and affective organization. I can't tell you what will happen a half year from now. He may be back on the streets; I certainly don't guarantee a thing.
>
> Turning now to the enrichment of normal sexual behaviour through the use of psychedelics...[266]

People who feel angry when they read these sort of comments should know that they are not alone.

Drugs of all types have also often been the instruments of oppression and experimentation of the truly 'mad scientist' type. The military are keen users of drugs for everything from keeping their own troops awake, reducing their sexual desire and poisoning the enemy.

For just these reasons we should never assume that a drug is *the* answer. Drugs are part of our social context, they and their effects are embedded within our lived in world. Were this not the case they would have no meaning, for good or ill, and would not be usable agents of transgression. But the inevitable social contextualisation need not mean that drug experience cannot be part of our project of self-discovery. For instance, the Nuremberg rallies of the Third Reich were quintessential ritual invocations of Mars, but this does not mean that we cannot use ritual and drama to change consciousness for aims that are not totalitarian. Nor does it mean that Mars is an 'evil' god. Indeed the very fact that the techniques of transgression can become the techniques of oppression should give us all the more reason to disseminate them across society. Only by developing an ongoing engagement and *ownership* of these techniques can individuals remain aware of, and oppose, forces in society that would seek to limit or impose a specific view of the universe. By owning these techniques of changing consciousness we are empowered to change our own minds and to be aware of when others are trying to change our minds for us. Being empowered with the technology of transgression keeps meaning in play and ensures that it does not become ossified. As an example; there is such a thing as fascist art, but that art seeks (as part of its 'deployment as a technology of Power') to dominate and drive out many other art forms as being 'impure'. By empowering people with the techniques and understanding of art they can understand what is going on, and may be in a stronger position to challenge it (both directly (through their own art) and indirectly (by the way in which they choose to internally read the message of the art).[267]

## Strength to Dream

That society, especially in industrialised and post-industrialised cultures, is in the throws of massive change today is axiomatic. Everywhere we can see the 'polymorphous perversity' of the post-modern explosion, the technocratic and humanitarian shock waves of modernity. In the arts a man cuts a cow in two and pickles it. Meanwhile, human genetic information is inserted into living bovines. As fast as commercialism reduces our cultural icons to sugary cartoon animation, so new international underground icons emerge.

Drugs experience informs and has informed our society, and with increasing potency since World War II. As drug culture has expanded, a number of interpretations of the position of drugs in our society vie with each other for Power. We have a 'War on Drugs', 'the chemical generation', the legalisation lobby, the 'just say no' discourse – many stories woven around the central spectre of drugs. The drug has become perhaps its own archetypal force; the modern philosopher's stone, the medicine and poison rolled into one multivocal symbol.

Movements such as rave culture, surrealism and street art often play with such 'archetypal' images, combining them in disconcerting, strange and whimsical ways. In this way art, like the transgressive use of drugs, opens our minds to the occult Other. In rave culture, drugs and art combine in a powerful synergy. No one who has attended a full-on Goa trance party (complete with ultraviolet banners of *Shiva Nataraja*; the dancing god) can fail to see the esoteric influence flowing into the room through the vision of the artists.

As well as having a science of drugs, our society also needs an art of their use. This recalls Aleister Crowley's definition of magic as being both an '..art and science'.

Many artistic movements (in the conventional sense), including those who seek to play with or distort our ideas about the world, do not overtly espouse the use of drugs (such as the surrealists, or the op-art movement). They might reject ideas that their work has any 'mystical' meaning, but these rejections do not invalidate this interpretation.[268] Artists, as Oliver Sacks points out, are 'the antennae of culture'.[269] If you want to find out 'what's hot' in culture, don't read books on philosophy, go to an art gallery, go and check out street art, observe how mainstream style changes and listen to the rumbles of the avant-garde underground. Art is a transgression. Art emerges from the transgressive act, in the rich borderland between ideas. It leads culture, creates it and destabilises it at the same time. Art is perhaps the most economically useless but culturally most significant human practice.

I believe that drugs, wisely used, can provide humanity with a new art. Another transgressive gateway to the realm of the liminal. I believe that drugs are an important way to renew and revive our global culture. A culture that legitimised the use of drugs would be a culture that did not fear change. A society that validated and encouraged transformative experience would be a 'spiritual' culture. It wouldn't be a static utopia with everything 'sorted'. Rather it would be an environment where individuals could move towards authenticity and self-actualisation - a society that was both challenged by, but also supportive of these goals.

## You Never Blow your Trip Forever

Drugs are themselves the Derridian 'trace' - the liminal locality between mind/body emotional/intellectual, inside/outside. They show us the futility of separating the universe into strict compartments of knowledge. They are both the 'pivot points' of duality and a questioning, an unpicking, of that very duality.

Much of what we consider separate (such as the idea of a 'normal' self and a 'supplemental' sense of the chemically altered, drug modified, 'I') is destabilised by the drug experience. Drugs force us to question the boundaries not only of the physical soma (where is the effect? In the drug, in my mind, or is it an emergent property, a synergy, between the two?) but, potentially, of all aspects of our being. Drugs *play* with the mind.

Of course we can deconstruct the world without drug experience. Take the example of the commonplace duality of emotions vs. intellect. The argument that emotions and intellectual ideas are two separate things may easily be deconstructed analytically. For instance an emotion can be described in logical terms – perhaps by psychoanalysis, psychology, neurology and put into an intellectual framework. Likewise an intellectual idea can be said to spring from a whole host of emotional effects. For instance I may be an intellectually committed Marxist because of my family history and emotional landscape as much as being intellectually convinced by theoreticians.[270] Drug experience might provide this type of expressible insight, the sort we can arrive at using deductive reasoning (itself a neurochemical experience?). Yet drugs can go beyond insight as we usually mean it.

What then do drugs, or rather what does the notion of an art of drug use, offer? In essence it offers us a technique, what Michael Harner calls (referring to shamanism as a whole) a 'technology of the sacred'. The use of drugs is one technology (or 'art') within the body of knowledge which I call magic. The knowledge drug experience can supply is not of a particular type (an expressible idea, concept or revelation – though it may be these things too) so much as it is knowledge of the Other – a portal of transgression. Drugs might not necessarily provide us with specific understanding or illumination. What they do is to demonstrate in real, practical terms the play of meaning and interpretation, to illuminate the Real landscape upon which the symbolic realm is based. They may lead to new inventions, new creeds, new orthodoxy but this is determined by how the experience is made meaningful (through the shamanic return).

The paradox is that knowledge of drugs is a way of using knowledge to reach the unknowable, Huxley's 'Mind at Large', the numinous, the 'Real' - call it what you like. We cannot resolve this paradox but only play in the meaningful and meaninglessness of it.

The process of learning (by drug experience or any other aspect of the autopoietic project) is the process of being supported by 'materials' (as Shulgin calls drugs) or 'teachers' through the dialectic between duality.

Human experience is the field of play (in the sense that Vygotsky, Derrida and Winnicott use the term). We live in a world not of fixed certainties but one in which meaning, perspective, power and destabilisation eternally play with and through each other. The educationalist Bruner expresses this when he says:

> When we enter human life, it is as if we walk on stage into a play whose enactment is already in progress – a play whose somewhat open plot determines what part we may play and towards what denouements we may be heading. Others on stage already have a sense of what the play is about, enough of a sense to make negotiation with a newcomer possible.[271]

The play of life, in Hindu mysticism, the dance of Maya, is something which intelligent drug use can help us to understand. It can shake us up and provide new perspectives which can be built into a weird and wonderful variety of symbolic structures or interpretations. As I said at the beginning of this book, these discoveries aren't limited to mystics. Here is chemist Albert Hofmann expressing his own understanding about the play of meaning through the world:

> Of greatest significance to me has been the insight that I attained as a fundamental understanding from all of my LSD experiments: what one commonly takes as "the reality", including the reality of one's own individual person, by no means signifies something fixed, but rather something that is ambiguous - that there is not only one, but that there are many realities, each comprising also a different consciousness of the ego.[272]

Of course reductionists may say that this 'flexibility of reality' is caused by poisoning, by derangement of the 'normal' chemical balances in the brain. Perhaps materialist science is right. Perhaps drug experience represents a warping of 'real' reality. But even if drug experience is delusion it teaches us this; although we may think we know the world we only do so through interpretation. There are many different interpretations of the world, perhaps some are better suited to some tasks than others. (What use would it be if an art critic only talked about the chemical composition of the paint used by an artist?) Drug experience can help shake us out of our conceptual complacency. Even those people who do not believe in magic can surely see the value in this.

I would not necessarily argue that Hofmann could not have come to his insights without drugs. What I would assert is that in order to learn *in any sense* we must pass through the liminal realm. The space between one current sense of Self and into the Other. In making our way across these zones of proximal development we need as much help as we can get.

Good teachers can show the way and for Hofmann, as for thousands of other people, drug experience has been a good teacher.

Drug experience can provide the opportunity to deeply explore the truth of the world. Experiences of being able to understand the birds whilst on fly agaric, to fly in the air with datura, to descend into the heart of the atom with ketamine – making sense of these things is a challenge. Moreover it is a necessity. We spend too much time, (in industrialised cultures at any rate) thinking that to be 'straight' is to be normal. If this is so, then why do we continually seek out the sharing of drugs to relax, to celebrate, to grieve? Whatever we decide to make of our drug experiences, the human spirit contains them, they are a real and significant aspect of human experience. To ignore them, their insights and difficulties, is like doing oceanography but never looking deeper than the first two inches below the sea's surface.

I believe that the learning, the transgressions that drugs can support us through, can provide a powerful medicine to help *make us become who we can be*. I would never deny the dangers and difficulties associated with exploring the self through drugs, no-one who has used drugs intelligently is unaware of how powerful these experiences can be. But I feel that we can consciously approach and engage with these powerful spirits. They may be just the teachers that our society needs, if only we can learn to listen.

# Notes

1. The liminal realm is akin to the 'temporary autonomous zone' of the anarchist philosopher Hakim Bey in *The Temporary Autonomous Zone, Ontological Anarchy, Poetic Terrorism*, Autonomedia, 1991. In another sense it is the space of the 'transitional object' in the child psychoanalysis of D.W.Winnicott *Playing and Reality*, Routledge, 1971. In mythic terms the liminal space is the magic circle 'the place that is not a place, in a time that is not a time, between the realm of humans and that of the gods'.

2. See Ann and Alexander Shulgin *PIHKAL (Phenethylamines I Have Known And Loved)*, Transform Press, 1991.

3. This text is currently available on the internet. See www.hyperreal.com.

4. Alan Watts, *The Joyous Cosmology*, Jonathan Cape Ltd, 1974.

5. As parapsychologist Serena Roney-Dougal points out, in *Where Science and Magic Meet*, Element, 1991, neurochemistry is an emerging science and is exceedingly complex. Indeed the use of specific terminology, as well as basic assumptions within the discipline, are yet to be firmly established within the corpus of knowledge.

6. The spelling of 'magick' was adopted by Aleister Crowley, for esoteric reasons and to differentiate the magic of the shaman from the trickery of the stage magician. However in this book I have used the common spelling 'magic'.

7. Probably the most famous definition is that given by Crowley 'Magick is the Science and Art of causing change to occur in conformity with Will'. See *Magick In Theory and Practice*, Routledge and Kegan Paul, 1983. Although this may seem a ludicrously broad definition Crowley is, in one sense, hinting at the universality and quasi-Taoist nature of what Magic is.

8. There are lots of names for this 'peak state', from 'Gnosis' – used by the occultist Pete Carroll, through to a '+4' or the 'oceanic experience' as described by Alexander & Ann Shulgin.

9. Since humans have a sense of individual project. Other beings, such as pigs and birch trees, may well have projects too but we cannot say if this is case since we are logically bound by the human-centred world-view. By a sense of project I mean an instinctual drive to engage in the process of making meaning (called by psychoanalysis 'epistomophilia'). However much we

push back the sense of Self there still remains a sense of Self. But this Self is one in a constant state of flux, since the very existence of the Self demands the changing of the Self. This desire to simultaneously *be* the Self and to *change* the Self, is the magical impulse in our species.

10  See Luigi Zoja *Drugs, Addiction and Initiation*, Sigo Press, 1989. The idea of a drug as a 'material' also begs the question where we place the limit of this term. A photon is physical, it is a 'material' (certainly materialists should acknowledge that *everything* is a material). Can we therefore say that a flashing strobe light (which can certainly alter consciousness) is a drug?

11  In hyperactive children some areas of 'normal' brain function are depressed. Giving them amphetamines chemically stimulates these areas, leading to a reduction in hyperactive behaviours and increased attention span.

12  For an extreme example of the variability of reactions to a given drug see the account of an experiment with a drug called 5-TOM in the Shulgins' *PIHKAL* op cit.

13  See *The Bach Flower Remedies Step by Step,* Judy Howard, C.W.Daniel, 1990.

14  The supplement in Derridas' work is the idea that something can be added to a thing that is neither part of it but is not not a part of it. So a dietary supplement is *added* to ones' diet, but is not itself *different* from that diet.

15  See *Soma: Divine Mushroom of Immortality*, Harcourt Brace Jovanovich, 1971.

16  For instance one internet account suggests a link between the effect of DMT and geographical conditions. The report suggests that DMT experiences tend to be easier near bodies of water, and more traumatic in deserts. Other drug effects may also be susceptible to such environmental conditions. Perhaps differences of altitude, humidity or other factors might have significant effects in how particular drugs operate.

17  Set and setting is a now commonly used phrase in context of psychedelic investigations. Set is the inner, cultural meaning, personal expectations and reactions to a drug experience, and setting is the environmental conditions in which the drug is taken.

18  See *Plants of the Gods* Richard Evans Schultes and Albert Hofmann, Healing Arts Press, 1992.

19  See M.Foucault, *The Order of Things*, Tavistock, 1970. In which Foucault quotes; 'A certain Chinese encyclopædia" in which animals are divided into such categories as;

A - Belonging to the Emperor

B - Embalmed

C - Tame

D - Sucking pigs

E - Sirens

F - Fabulous

G - Stray dogs

H - Included in the present classification.

K - drawn with a very fine camel hair brush

L – etc.

M - having just broken a water picture.'

20 Crowley's *777 & Other Qabalistic Writings* (Samuel Weiser, 1986) provides a method for symbolically linking together every aspect of the universe in qualitative, poetic terms. This system of correspondences is fundamental to the western occult tradition. It provides 'chains of thought' which can be used to explore the relationships between apparently quite dissimilar groups of ideas. In fact humans engage in this practice of association all the time. As an example consider what *colour* different forms of music are. Perhaps purple might be heavy metal, brown for folk, and maybe blue for 'the blues'. The aim is not to have a fixed set of correspondences but to explore the permutations and relationships that can be found between concepts.

21 The 'qabalistic sephira' is a qualitative category for different forces in the universe. The names given are the Hebrew names as they appear on the Tree of Life. For example, Kether means 'Crown', Binah 'Understanding', and Yesod 'Foundation'. Note how some attributions by Crowley are not drugs in the usual sense of the word (e.g. 'corn' for Malkuth). Anhalonium Lewinii is mescaline.

22 For instance peyote which 'is the footprints of the little deer' or Ololiuqui which is the 'vine of the serpent'.

23 As Paracelsus points out, the difference between poison and medicine is one of dose, but it is also dependent on one's perspective of what a drug *is*. For example peyote often makes users ill. In American shamanism the vomiting that accompanies the drug experience is called 'getting well' rather than getting sick, and is seen as the mind and body cleansing itself.

24  The use of the term 'trip' is one that I particularly like since it emphasises the experiential nature of the human relationship with drugs. It implies a journey, a 'travelling without moving' as novelist Frank Herbert would put it. The term also has overtones of the shamanic journey or flight. Ethnographer Kenneth M. Kensinger in *Banisteriopsis Usage Among the Peruvian Cashinahua* mentions that the Cashinahua also use a word which translates very closely to 'trip' when speaking of their shamanic hallucinatory journeys. See *Hallucinogens and Shamanism*, Michael Harner (ed) Oxford University Press 1973.

25  Snyder, S.H. et al, 'Drugs, Neurotransmitters, and Schizophrenia' pp.1243-1253. Hollister, L.E.. 'Drug-Induced Psychoses and Schizophrenic Reactions: A Critical Comparison' *Annals of New York Academy of Sciences*, 1962, 96:80-92.

26  Foucault, although clearly acknowledging that many artists go 'mad' does not himself attribute their art as a function of their madness. 'The madness of Nietzsche, the madness of Van Gogh or of Artaud, belongs to their work perhaps neither more nor less profoundly, but in quite another way...And yet this frequency must be taken seriously, as if it were the insistence of a question: from the time of Hölderlin and Nerval, the number of writers, painters, and musicians who have 'succumbed' to madness has increased; but let us make no mistake here; between madness and the work of art, there has been no accommodation...Artaud's madness does not slip through the fissures of the work of art; his madness is precisely the *absence of the work of art*...Van Gogh, who did not want to ask "permission from doctors to paint pictures', knew quite well that his work and his madness were incompatible...*where there is a work of art, there is no madness*".' Michel Foucault, *Madness and Civilisation*, Random House, 1965.

27  See R. Silverberg, *Drug Themes in Science Fiction*, US Government National Institute of Drug Abuse, 1973.

28  Unlike say in the Japanese Kabuki theatre where artificiality is seen as beautiful. As the great 18th century onnagata (Kabuki actor who plays female roles) Yoshizawa Ayame declared woman could not herself express ideal feminine beauty, 'for she could only rely on her physical characteristics, and therefore not express the synthetic ideal'.

29  See Timothy Leary *The Politics of Ecstasy*, Ronin Publishing, 1997 (reprint).

30  See Dion Fortune, *Psychic Self-Defence*, Aquarian, 1967. Fortune argues that the use of drugs in magic is dangerous and undesirable as well as illegal.

31  Shulgin in *PHIKAL* (op cit.) for an excellent discussion of natural vs. synthetic drugs see p 236.

32  Although now a dated term, 'rave' conveys the recreation and potentially transgressive use of MDMA in dance culture better than any other.

33  '...these "intoxicants", which nowadays are used to produce mere excitement or brutal drunkenness, were at first looked upon as media able to rise the mere man up to a level with his gods, and enable him to communicate with them, as was certainly the case with the "soma" of the Hindu ecstatics and the hashish I have seen used by some tribes of Arabs.' Dr J.W. Kingsley Personal letter to Captain Bourke, 1888.

34  Professor Mircea Eliade in *Shamanism* first published in 1951 claims that drug use in shamanism is '...only a vulgar substitute for pure trance...an imitation of the state which the shaman is no longer capable of attaining otherwise'. As I show the distinction between drug/non-drug visionary experience is a moot point. Moreover ethnographic experience, especially in the Americas would certainly seem to challenge Eliade's view, as do writers such as R.G. Wasson in Peter T Furst (Ed), *Flesh of the Gods* London 1972.

35  As demonstrated by a whole host of western occult practice, including classic grimoires (texts of magical operations) such as *The Sacred Magic of Abra Melin the Mage* and the *Goetia*..

36  Once more we see the Derridian *trace* in action in that science, the belief system that replaced 'superstition', and eventually religion, grew out of the occult world view. If we name some important figures that the discourse of science deems to be important we find Pythagoras, the mathematical mystic, Dr John Dee occultist and writer of the preface for the first English translation of Euclid, Giordano Bruno engineer and magician and of course Isaac Newton who wrote more on astrology and religious metaphysics than anything else.

37  The story of Henry Durbin (who may warrant the title of the world's first parapsychologist) is the focus for a forthcoming paper by Eddie Marcus and Helen Gray 'Keeping Possession; The politics of reason and witchcraft in 18th century Bristol'.

38  See *A History of Witchcraft, Sorcerers, Heretics and Pagans*, Jeffery B. Russell, Thames and Hudson, 1980. Though the work of Eddie Marcus and Helen Gray challenges this assumption.

39  Helen Gray & Eddie Marcus *Keeping Possession* op cit.

40  See Montague Summers preface to *Malleus Mallificarum* (1928) in which he likens witches to the 'anarchists, nihilists and Bolsheviks'. The title 'witch' was also adopted by feminist groups, particularly in the USA in the 1960s, see Jeffrey B.Russell, op cit.

41  Current Halloween traditions are an excellent example of a revised tradition the impetus of which has come predominately into British society. If nothing else this serves to remind adults that children too are part of society and wield their own power.

42  For examples of the modern cultural fear of physical liminal space see Duerr op cit.

43  A common motif in the folktales collected by the brothers Grimm.

44  There are many different forms of these rituals. See Hans Peter Duerr, *Dreamtime: concerning the boundary between wilderness and civilization*. Basil Blackwell, 1985.

45  'As late as the Middle Ages, the witch was still the *hagazussa*, a being that sat on the *Hag*, the fence, which passed behind the gardens and separated the village from the wilderness. She was a being who participated in both worlds. As we might say today, she was semi-demonic. In time, however, she lost her double features and evolved more and more into a representation of what was being expelled from culture, only to return, distorted, in the night.' Duerr *ibid*.

46  Such as the disturbingly surreal abode of the witch Baba Yaga.

47  As evidenced by the research of Henry Durbin and the work of Montague Summers.

48  See *Enemies of God*, John Hopkins University Press, 1981.

49  Johnson, on the mysterious disappearance of witches is quoted by H.Luventhal, *In the Shadow of the Enlightenment* (New York University Press, 1976). 'No sir, witchcraft had ceased; and therefore an act of parliament was passed to prevent prosecution for what was not witchcraft. Why it ceased, we cannot tell, as we cannot tell the manner of many other things'.

50  See Catherine Summers & Julian Vayne, *Seeds of Magick*, Foulsham, 1990.

51  Duerr *op. cit*.

52  Duerr *ibid*.

53  See Albert Goldman *Disco*, Hawthorn Books, 1978

54  Some writers, notably George Bataille argue that the transgressive, ultimately, re-enforces 'Law' in the world. This is a very technical argument but suffice it to say that if transgression gives rise to society, which in turn gives rise to Law, then it could equally be said that Law itself provides the opportunity to transgress since it draws lines in the cultural sand and, by doing so, delineates both the sacred and profane, and thus makes the transgressive possible.

55  See my article 'Turn On, Tune In, Break Out' in *Talking Stick Magazine* 1991.

56  Although the link between hashish and 'reefer madness' has always been a strong one in the minds of those attempting to dissuade people from using the drug, it seems to have little foundation. Although it may be true that the Thuggee smoked dope, that may simply be because *everyone* smoked dope in these cultures. What is perhaps interesting is how this, generally, most languid of intoxicants came to be linked with violence.

57  The confusion between what might be called the 'social effect' of drugs and their 'inherent effects' is neatly analysed by Lester Grinspoon in *Marihuana Reconsidered* (Harvard University Press, 1971). In this apologia for cannabis use, Grinspoon points out that the aphrodisiac properties of marijuana are better thought of as a general relaxing of inhibitions. In this way marijuana acts much like alcohol. It does not, in itself, cause sexual arousal or any other assumed manifestation of 'reefer madness'. 'The user [of cannabis] may say things that he ordinarily would not, but in general will not do things that are foreign to his nature. If he is not a criminal, he will not usually commit a crime.'

58  Of course this could be a joke or he may have forgotten what he really meant to say...

59  See Robert Sabbag *Snowblind* Pan Books, 1979.

60  See Bruce Eisner, *Ecstasy: The MDMA Story*, Ronin Publishing, 1989.

61  *The Hashish Club* translated by Ralph Gladstone *Marijuana Papers* 1972

62  See Eisner *op cit*.

63  For this well spring is outside of reason and language. It is the Wittgensteinian 'unspeakable', a concept (albeit appearing in different guises) common to the works of Bataille, Nietzsche, Hegel and others.

64  See Ann & Alexander Shulgin *TIHKAL* Transform Press, 1997 p.174.

65 Babalon, in Crowley's 'Thelemic' cosmology represents one aspect of the 'primordial feminine archetype'. Babalon is a goddess, a metaphysical representation of the 'yin' of Oriental thought.

66 John B. Watson 'Psychology as the Behaviourist Views It', see *Modern Philosophy of the Mind*, David Berman (Ed) Everyman, 1995. Of course the project of excluding consciousness from any research is doomed from the start, since presumably Watson is a conscious entity attempting to communicate his ideas to other conscious minds.

67 See Maslow characteristics of self-actualizers, which include 'peak experiences', *Motivation and Personality*, Harper and Row, 1970 and Czikszentmihalyi (1975)

68 In the sense that Sartre and other 20th century philosophers use this term. Crowley calls the project of being authentic, the practice of finding and doing one's 'True Will'.

69 See Abraham Maslow's 'hierarchy of needs'. Growth is, *in itself*, a rewarding, and exciting process. {Examples include} the fulfilling of yearnings and ambitions, like that of being a good doctor; the acquisition of skills, like playing the violin or being a good carpenter; the steady increase of understanding about people or about the universe, or about oneself; the development of creativeness in whatever field; or, most importantly, simply the ambition to be a good human being...It is simply inaccurate to speak in such instances of tension-reduction, implying thereby getting rid of an annoying state. For these states are not annoying (Maslow 1968).

70 Current education policy in many industrialised nations, including the UK, favours the notion of learning as the acquisition of competence. This is a pragmatic, capitalist, but hugely impoverished view of learning generally, and education in particular.

71 'Self-actualization is idiosyncratic, since every person is different...The individual [must do] what *he*, individually, is fitted for. A musician must make music, an artist must paint, a poet must write, if he is to be ultimately at peace with himself. What a man *can* be, he *must* be.' Maslow, *Towards a Psychology of Being* (2nd ed) Harper & Row, 1968.

72 Personally I think evolution is a believable theory, though by no means the complete answer to the question 'why are living things the way they are'. If nothing else neo-Darwinians tend to demonstrate the same 'Catch 22' devotion to their 'meta-narrative' as religious zealots or Marxists and I'm distrustful of that sort of belief system.

73  Note the internalisation of thought may give rise to language as a means to express this, see Nicholas Humphrey, *A History of the Mind,* Vintage, 1993

74  Animal experiments might be interesting and even useful, but would it be moral to do experiments on say Jews, black people or single mothers? The question is a moral one, not simply about the fruitfulness of research. As I will show much drug experience is mental and there are only so many questions we can ask, or get useful answers from if our subject is a rat. Science does have a disreputable history of putting research and technique before human needs, and certainly before the needs of other species of the biosphere considered as a whole. In a human context the many tens of thousands of full frontal lobotomies performed in the US and UK alone stand as testimony to this.

75  The brain is a 'high resolution' system. This means that we will try to make sense of even 'random' things by giving them meaning. This is one answer to the question why do we see recognisable shapes in clouds (or indeed images of the Madonna on Mars).

76  Daniel Dennett's term for the 'black box' marked 'consciousness' which often gets slyly slipped into cognitive scientific descriptions of the mind. As he rightly asserts this is just an example of pushing the problem backwards, by suggesting that within the brain there is an area that 'decodes' information and makes ideas. This just re-states the problem and goes nowhere near addressing just what that 'area' is.

77  Though the ubiquitous alcohol and the most powerful naturally occurring psychedelic *Salvia divinorum* seem to work through different mechanisms.

78  See (amongst many others) Geschwind, N. & Galaburda, A.M. *Cerebral Lateralization,* Bradford, 1987.

79  See the paper (originally published in 1981) 'Brain and Mind in Desana Shamanism', in *Rainforest Shamans,* Gerardo Reichel-Dolmatoff, Green Books, 1997.

80  See Reichel-Dolmatoff *ibid.*

81  The *ajna chakra,* in Indian occultism, is the place of 'clear seeing'. Magical powers such as clairvoyance is attained when this chakra is opened..

82  By converting serotonin into n-acetylserotonin in the dark pinealocyte.

83  Monoamine oxidase (MAO) inhibitors block the activity of an enzyme that can destroy both norepinephrine and serotonin. In this way MAO inhibitors increase the concentration of these neurotransmitters. These

inhibitors (which include the commercial anti-depressants phenelzine or Nardil) are dangerous in that, if taken with a drug that effects serotonin function such as LSD or MDMA, they can lead to a hypertensive crisis (increased heart rate, blood pressure and possible eventual collapse). In theory a carefully controlled balance of, say MDMA and an MAO inhibitor could increase both the high and duration of a trip. However experiments in striking the chemical balance would be difficult and maybe fatal (there are some scary internet accounts that I've read from brave/ stupid people experimenting with the MAO/MDMA cocktail). In theory a similar effect should be observed if tricyclic antidepressants (which prevent serotonin and norepinephrine reuptake) were combined with a serotonin effecting psychedelic. Tricyclics on the market include Imipramine (Tofranil) but again experimentation should be undertaken with caution.

84 See *Food of the Gods*, Terence McKenna, Rider, 1992.

85 'Anthropological studies suggests that epileptics, and those we label as psychotic, are often chosen for training as shamans, since they are held by their illness to be linked in some special way with the world of spirits and psi abilities.' See Serena Roney-Dougal *op cit*.

86 That is between mind and body.

87 The production of 5-MeO-DMT *in vivo* in the pineal gland, along with work by Serena Roney-Dougal (*op cit*) and the paper *The Pineal Gland, LSD and Serotonin* (Russ McClay, 1976) support this suggestion.

88 See 'Psybermagick', *Chaos International* & *Asafoetida*, 1995.

89 Genetic factors can certainly be important in our descriptions of what it means to be human, but they are far from determining factors. The rush to patent genetic code is certainly part of the financial support provided to genetic researchers.

90 For an insight into this condition see the film *Rain Man*.

91 Lightning speed calculation is sometimes encountered in people with other neurological disability. See Oliver Sacks, *The Man Who Mistook his Wife for a Hat*, HarperCollins (3rd ed), 1990.

92 Thanks to Helen and Sara (who have both worked with people with autism) for pointing out this little phenomena which is rarely mentioned in the literature on the subject.

93 See *Schizophrenia The Facts*, Ming T. Tsuang, OUP, 1982.

94  See *Drugs for Mental Illness*, Lickey and Marvin, W.H.Freeman and Company, 1983.

95  *Ibid.*

96  I've seen and heard of this behaviour a number of times. Datura is a powerful drug. The experience that it produces can such a high degree of what virtual reality designers call 'presence' (i.e. little or no sense of illusion, of being aware that you are tripping, is felt), that users may simply feel no social inappropriateness in going naked. In a comfortable environment removing your clothes whilst using psychedelics may provide a certain sense of freedom and comfort. Perhaps this explains the archetypal nakedness of 1960s acid-popping hippies, and the 'skyclad' rituals of witches (both ancient and modern).

97  Drugs for Mental Illness *op cit.*

98  See Crowley *Magick In Theory and Practice*, Routledge and Kegan Paul, 1983.

99  Tsuang, *op cit.*

100 Solo artist and lead vocalist and songwriter of *The Throwing Muses*.

101 The paediatrician and psychoanalyst D.W.Winnicott writes, 'It is important for us that we find clinically *no sharp line* between health and the schizoid state or even between health and full-blown schizophrenia'. (*Playing and Reality,* Routledge, 1971). Madness, in its many forms exists as part of a continuum. Indeed perhaps the greater part of any madness is culturally constructed, as Foucault points out in *Madness and Civilization* (Random House, 1965), '...it is not surprising to find the eighteenth century nosographers often classifying vertigo as madness, and more rarely hysterical convulsions; this is because it is often impossible to find in hysterical convulsions the unity of language, while vertigo affords the delirious affirmation that the world is really 'turning around.' Such delirium is a necessary and sufficient reason for a disease to be called madness.'

102 In *Sanity Madness and the Family* by Laing and Emerson (1964), they put forward the important view that schizophrenia is 'a form of violence perpetrated by some people against others'. Laing later developed the view that schizophrenia is 'itself a natural way of healing our own appalling state of alienation called normality'. And that, 'madness need not be all breakdown...it may also be breakthrough'. As Bateson points out, the 'patient embarks on a voyage of discovery (death) and returns (rebirth) to the normal world with new insights. Schizophrenia in this way is considered

a natural process by some psychologists, a voyage into "inner space" ' (through the liminal into 'the other'), a 'natural healing process'. Laing argues that the natural course of schizophrenia is rarely allowed to happen because we are too busy *treating* the patient. I would agree with this inasmuch as the treatment (or support, or 'set and setting') for schizophrenia is inappropriate. If nothing else imagine being on acid in a Victorian mental asylum, not knowing when (if ever) your trip was going to end. Much as gynaecology and obstetrics have slowly come around to the idea that pregnancy and birth is not a disease, so perhaps it would be better to move to a view of schizophrenia as a difficult and challenging process that people can be helped and supported through. Certainly this may require the use of therapeutic techniques that are used at present, but the way they are used and why needs to come under serious scrutiny.(See *Psychology* Richard D.Gross Hodder & Stoughton 1992 p952)

103 See Dr Simon Baron-Cohen and Dr Patrick Bolton, *Autism - the Facts*, OUP, 1993.

104 Timothy Taylor *The Prehistory of Sex,* Fourth Estate, 1996.

105 Dr Simon Baron-Cohen and Dr Patrick Bolton *op cit.*

106 The exact method of LSD's function in the brain is still unclear. The most commonly advanced theory is that the LSD molecule, which structurally resembles that of the neurotransmitter serotonin, mimics the effect of serotonin in the synapse and over stimulates the neurones. Of course this does not address the reason why (in either a neurochemical or philosophical sense) LSD can generate such profound changes in awareness.

107 See for instance 'The Psychedelic Model of Schizophrenia: The Case of N,N-Dimethyltryptamine' by Gillin, Kaplan, Stillman & Wyatt *American Journal of Psychiatry* 133;2 pp.203-208, February 1976

The Abstract for this paper reads:

The authors review the research on N,N-dimethyltryptamine (DMT) as a possible 'schizotoxin'. DMT produces psychedelic effects when administered to normal subjects, the means are present to synthesize it in man, it has occasionally been found in man, and tolerance to its behavioural effects is incomplete. However, DMT concentrations have not been proven to differ significantly in schizophrenics and normal controls. Also, in vivo synthesis of DMT has not been convincingly demonstrated, and the psychological changes it produces do not closely mimic the symptoms of schizophrenia. The authors conclude that more data are necessary before the validity of this theory can be determined.

108  See, amongst other examples, *The Illustrated Book of Herbs*, Sarah Bunney (ed.), Octopus, 1987.

109  Ross et al 1987, also current internet resources on the treatment of autism.

110  Richard Gross *op cit*

111  *Ibid*

112  Although highly simplified, the principle of cerebral lateralisation is used with dramatic effect by Betty Edwards in her book *Drawing on the Left Hand Side of the Brain* (Fontana, 1979) in teaching art skills. The impressive results of her training, using ideas drawn from lateralisation studies, speak for themselves.

113  I agree that amphetamine psychosis is close to the symptoms of severe schizophrenia. However I believe that it is primarily the anxiety that amphetamine-type stimulation induces (whether through drug use or endogenous dopamine changes) which leads to the patient to be unable to cope with the LSD/serotonin like effects of the condition itself. Treating the anxiety and relieving the major symptoms is an excellent start, but by no means is it a cure.

114  Objections to drug therapy include 1) it treats symptoms not basic problems, 2) it dulls the patient so they cannot communicate effectively, and 3) it is a cheap, quick-fix solution.

115  Marvin E.Lickley, Barbara Gordon *op cit*.

116  Daniel Dennett *Consciousness Explained,* Penguin, 1991.

117  See *Can We Solve the Mind-Body Problem?* in *Modern Philosophy of the Mind*, David Berman (Ed), 1995.

118  See Colin Blakemore, *The Mind Machine,* Penguin, 1994.

119  How we know that something is intelligent in itself is a philosophical issue, discussed at length by Dennett (*ibid*). For most purposes I am happy with proposed criteria from the inventor of the computer Alan Turing. Namely, can I communicate with the computer (perhaps through a keyboard) and be convinced that the responses I am getting could well be coming from a human? Interestingly, though often overlooked when Turin is being quoted by materialists, Turin also asks that an artificial intelligence be able to demonstrate the type of telepathic and psychic ability which humans are capable of. See *Alan Turing: the Enigma,* Random House, 1992.

120  See the analysis of this match reported in *Fortean Times* Issue 103 by Dave Walsh

121  See the Culture novels of Iain M.Banks.

122  See *Bright Air, Brilliant Fire,* Gerald Edelman, HarperCollins 1992.

123  See Jay Stevens, *Storming Heaven; LSD and the American Dream,* Paladin, 1989.

124  There is a feedback loop between sunlight and endocrine systems mediated by the pineal gland. This factor has been identified as perhaps being significant in paranormal events and other altered states by Serena Roney-Dougal and others.

125  This fact is recognised by even the most conservative writers on drugs. In *Heroin today: commodity, consumption, control and care* by ISDD Research and Development Unit (in *A Land Fit for Heroin?* Edited by Nicholas Dorn and Nigel South, MacMillian 1987). The authors write …injection carries certain symbolic aspects (though these may vary from group to group), and not only the users themselves but also non-users aware of their practice may react to injectors in specific ways that mark them off from 'the normal'. Thus the mode of administration may have consequences for how users perceive themselves and their drug use, and hence consequences for their future use: some injectors may become quite involved in playing at the role of 'addict'.

126  See Bruce Eisner *op cit.*.

127  In *Consciousness Explained* Dennet tries to show that it is paradoxical (and therefore unpleasantly dualistic) to assume that the brain and mind are made of different stuff. '…there is only one sort of stuff, namely *matter* – the physical stuff of physics, chemistry, and physiology – and the mind is somehow nothing but a physical phenomena. In short, the mind is the brain'. However the interactionalist approach that I support argues that the material world itself shows just such paradoxical findings as those Dennet rails against. For example the wave/particle duality of light and the 'top down' lessons we can learn from looking at the placebo and other pharmacological effects.

128  A good example of the genes-environment interaction is that of the disease phenylketonuria (PKU), which involves the inheritance of two recessive genes which prevent the body secreting an enzyme, whose function is to metabolise phenylalanine (a common constituent of many foods, especially dairy produce). If untreated phenylalanine builds up and eventually poisons the nervous system, causing severe mental retardation, and,

eventually death. However by putting the baby on a low-protein diet (for the first 10-12yrs) these effects can be prevented and normal IQ will develop. This suggests that talk of low or high IQ genes is flawed since the genes depend upon the environment in which they express themselves. In themselves they are neither bright nor dull.

129  See Antionio R. Damasio *Descartes' Error*, Picador 1996.

130  See Andrew Tyler *Street Drugs,* Hodder & Stoughton 1995 and Nicholas Saunders *Ecstasy and the Dance Culture,* 1995

131  Lynn Zimmer & John P.Morgan *Marijuana Myths, Marijuana Facts,* Lindesmith Centre 1997

132  This effect is quite common. As an example see Ann Shulgin's account in *TIHKAL* p 45 *op cit.*

133  See Alexander and Ann Shulgin *op cit.*

134  See Peter Redgrove *The Black Goddess and the Sixth Sense*, Paladin, 1987.

135  See Thoman Nagel, 'What is it Like to be a Bat?' in *Modern Philosophy of the Mind* (op cit).

136  Though this is a slightly different use of the term autism it still applies to an individual who has not yet crossed the imaginative discontinuity.

137  See Dollores LaChapelle, *Sacred Land, Sacred Sex, Rapture of The Deep,* Finn Hill Arts, 1988.

138  We could also legitimately describe the neurological aspects of the learning process in terms of chemical experiences, such as changes in glycol activity in the brain.

139  Investigated by both Freud and Lacan.

140  Note how taboo means both sacred and forbidden.

141  For an excellent discussion of taboo breaking transgression in the context of the tantric cults see *Kali, The Black Goddess of Dakshineswar* by Elizabeth U. Harding, Nicholas-Hays 1993 p.72.

142  McKenna, in typically poetic terms described the shaman as one who has seen 'the wiring under the board', a person who has 'been to the end' (though McKenna's emphasis on eschatology, perhaps necessarily, has more in common with a post-Christian than archaic world view.

143  Gender is itself a much more mutable category than the pragmatic male/female dimorphism usually adopted. The post-modern break-up of gender boundaries, the adoption of terms such as 'fluid' to designate

sexual desire (rather than homosexual, heterosexual, bisexual) has served to illustrate this. Even at a physical level our ideas of gender are subject to destabilisation. As an example of this there are children born with normal female genitalia who, at about 12 years of age, their vaginas heal over, two testicles descend and they grow full-size penises. See *Report on the Batista Family* by Imperato-McGinley, J., Guerro, L., Gautier, T & Peterson, R.E., 'Steroid 5-reductase deficiency in man: An Inherited form of male pseudohermaphroditism'. *Science, 186, 1213-16.*

144   See Edmund Husserl, *Ideas*, Collier, 1962.

145   See, amongst his works, Arthur Koestler *The Ghost in the Machine*, 1967.

146   See the strange case of the 'MDMA spectacles' (in the present work) in context of MDMA hallucinations.

147   Indeed some psychologists refer to this phenomena as 'macho ingestion syndrome'. Evolutionists have attempted to make sense of this phenomena. For a dubious, though certainly interesting interpretation of drug use in evolutionary terms see Colin Blakemore (op cit) and Jared Diamond, *The Rise and Fall of the Third Chimpanzee*, Vintage, 1991.

148   Some shamanic cultures that use hallucinogens (for example, the Jivaro Indians of Ecuador) consider datura to be a powerful way of contacting the spirit realm but 'too strong' to allow the shaman to operate in both worlds simultaneously (i.e. to perform magic). Michael Harner points out that to use drugs such as henbane, datura or belladona (often plants of the solanaceous order – i.e. the potato family) in north-west European folk shamanism (as reported in connection with European Witchcraft) may have resulted in the separate development of spell casting and ritual without the use of drugs (unlike in many south American shamanic cultures). The reason for this is that trying to hold together any sense of intentionality (whether it be to heal, curse or simply speak) under the influence of these drugs is extremely difficult. The visionary intoxication is simply too intense. See 'Hallucinogens in European Witchcraft' by Michael Harner in *Hallucinogens and Shamanism* op cit.

149   See Luigi Zoja op cit.

150   See Kenneth Grant, *Aleister Crowley and the Hidden God*, Muller, 1973. See also Louis T.Culling, *The Complete Magick Curriculum of the Secret Order G.B.G.*, Llewellyn, 1969, and *A Manual of Sex Magick*, Llewellyn, 1971.

151   See J.G.Bourke's 'Scatological Rites of All Nations' translated by Terence Deakin *in Drugs and Sexuality* David Solomon and George Andrews (Eds), Panther Books, 1973.

152 See Peter Redgrove op cit.

153 Longevity is certainly one of the aims of Tantrism, particularly the (arguably) more patriarchal Oriental Tantras, this magical benefit is generally seen as a side-effect of the Tantrik life style rather than the goal of it. For a broad analysis of Tantrism in a modern occult context see Katon Shual, *Sexual Magick*, Mandrake, 1995.

154 The term 'drug' still maintains a pragmatic meaning in language but we must remain clear that the boundaries of that term are always shifting, always becoming destabilised.

155 According to Terence McKenna, op cit.

156 For instance transgression using the sweat lodge or the Sun Dance ceremonies.

157 Once more we must not let 'temporal fascism' get the better of us. We really have no reason to assume, as McKenna does, that people in the past were too stupid to maintain a supply of soma for technological reasons. It is much more likely to have been a cultural *choice* arrived at by a whole variety of factors.

158 See the fascinating account of a 'high dose 2-CB trip' by Gracie and Zarkov archived at www.hyperreal.com (reproduced in these endnotes).

159 Perhaps by chemically sensitising the body/mind to pain transgressive rituals involving physical ordeals (such as S/M sex or other practices) could be heightened but without the need for increased physical damage to the organism.

160 See Dollores LaChapelle, op cit.

161 Though I would rather not completely exclude the possibility *a priori*.

162 The term unconscious mind is something of a catch all. My own understanding of the word and use of the term is informed by the psychoanalytical writing of Jung, and the occult work of Austin Osman Spare.

163 The fabled 'alien autopsy' of the Roswell alien.

164 See internet accounts of DMT use and my own overview of DMT in the present work.

165 Boszormenyi and Szara reported that schizophrenics do show diminished responsiveness to DMT, this may result from increased metabolism or variable tolerance resulting from long-term endogenous synthesis of DMT. See Boszormenyi A, Szara S; 'Dimethyltryptamine experiments

with psychotics', *Journal of Mental Science* 104;445-453, 1958. As already pointed out, schizophrenia is by no means exactly replicated by drug states, but the two do share some features. This research fits with the pattern in that schizophrenic people who spend more time in a SuperReal world should find psychedelics less potent but only slightly so.

166 See *Fortean Times* 108:25.

167 This is a term which I feel is more appropriate than the term 'visualisation' which is often used in esoteric literature. See Catherine Summers & Julian Vayne, *The Inner Space WorkBook*, Capall Bann, 1994.

168 See Catherine Summers & Julian Vayne, *Seeds of Magick* 1991.

169 For instance that magical gesture of 'The Rending of the Veil', see Crowley's *Magick in Theory and Practice* op cit.

170 For instance the invocation of Papa Legba (the Voudou god of the crossroads) which must be made at the start of any ritual to 'open up the ways' for the deities to manifest. Equally in western ritual magic the 'guardians of the watchtowers' of each cardinal direction are invoked to protect and empower the magic circle.

171 See Phil Hine *Walking Between the Worlds – techniques of modern shamanism*, Pagan News Publications, 1989.

172 See *Seeds of Magick*

173 The suggestion that 'the gods' are both symbolic ideas and also real, objective powers in the universe is one of the most commonly paradoxical views of western occultism. See, amongst others, Gerald J.Schueler, *Enochian Magic*, Llewellyn, 1988.

174 For a discussion on the relationship of the symbolic and the Real (in esoteric terms) see *Seeds of Magick*..

175 Flying experiences in shamanism are legion. How much is 'cultural', and how much might be the 'chemical' effect of certain drugs is debatable. For example the experience of flying was common to a group of volunteers given the shamanic brew yagé by Claudio Naranjo - see *Psychological Aspects of the Yage Experience in an Experimental Setting*, in *Hallucinogens and Shamanism*, op cit.

176 See, amongst others, Duerr op cit..

177 That is using 'organised imagination' to move what Castenada calls ones 'assemblage point' (sense of 'I') into the body of another creature. One

might equally use the term possession for this practice but I prefer the term 'borrowing' from the writing of Terry Pratchett.

178  See Crowley *Magick in Theory and Practice* op cit..

179  In the esoteric writing of the artist/magician Austin Osman Spare his formulation of magic is concerned with imaging the world 'as if' certain relationships exist (for example between a talisman and the person whom it is designed to protect). Whether this relationship is 'true' is not an answerable or useful question for Spare since most of what we experience in the symbolic realm is a 'lie' (day-to-day reality is much more based on 'as if' assumptions than the truth/falsehood dichotomy we usually imagine it to be). Spare's work is highly obtuse but he remains one of the most important esoteric writers (as well as a fine artist) of the 20th century.

180  See Israel Regardie, *The Golden Dawn*, Llewellyn, 1989 and others. The 'key scales' used to analyse the colours appearing in 'astral journeys' or 'pathworkings' can be found in Crowley *777*, and *The Book of Thoth*, Weiser 1980.

181  As John C. Lilly points out in 'If one is to explore the *unknown* one should take the minimum amount of baggage and not load one's self down with conceptual machinery which cannot be flexibly reoriented to accept and investigate the *unknown*...To remain sceptical of even this [i.e. Lilly's own model of the mind] formalization of this particular human computer's approach to this region is desirable. One does not over-value this particular approach; one looks for alternative approaches for exploratory purposes.' See *The Human Biocomputer* Abacus 1967.

182  W.Mrsich, *Erfahrungen mit Hexen und Hexensalbe* 1957.

183  Op cit.

184  A 'magical formula' is a qualitative statement about the relationship between specific elements in the symbolic realm that underlies a real pattern in the world. These formulae are expressed in highly symbolic terms, often in Qabalistic ciphers such as IAO, LAShTAL, IPSOS etc (where each Latin character is the transliteration of a Hebrew letter which is itself a 'multivocal symbol'). See, amongst others, Crowley, *Magick in Theory and Practice*.

185  See, amongst others, Kenneth Grant op cit.

186  Although he couched his work in an explicitly esoteric garb, Spare's work follows the thoughts of many other artists. 'The painter who likes to paint trees, becomes a tree. Children carry within them a natural drug...All

children possess the magic power of being able to change themselves into what they wish. Poets, in whom childhood is prolonged, suffer a great deal when they lose this power. This is undoubtedly one of the reasons which drives the poet to use opium...' – See *Opium*, Jean Cocteau.

187  Quoted in R.E.L.Masters and J.Houston, *The Varieties of Psychedelic Experience*, New York 1966.

188  Duerr op cit.

189  See Antonio Melechi's article 'Sense and Sensibility' in *Fortean Times* 113 august 1998.

190  See also Shulgin's *PIHKAL* p123 op cit.

191  Remember autistic people who live outside the imaginative realm have the sense that non-autistic people use telepathy to communicate. In a pragmatic sense this is true, since the imaginary realm constitutes a real dimension of linguistic meaning.

192  An amazing story was related in the December 1997 edition of the *British Medical Journal*. It concerned a woman who started hearing voices. Initially the woman (referred to as AB) heard one voice which told her not to be afraid, that it was a friend and wanted to help. AB sought medical advice and was treated by a consultant psychiatrist who said that she appeared to be cured after receiving medication and counselling. While on holiday the phenomena recurred, this time with two voices. The voices told AB to return to England immediately because there was something wrong with her brain. Once in London the voices provided her with an address which turned out to be the brain scan department of a large London hospital. The voices informed AB that she had an inflamed brain stem, and that she had a tumour. Mr Azuonye, of the mental health unit of Lambeth Healthcare NHS Trust decided to conduct a brain scan on AB, despite the fact that she had no symptoms of either problem. Although his colleagues criticised him for pandering to the delusions of AB the scan was performed and the result showed that AB did indeed have the illnesses she had identified. The tumour was successfully removed after which AB reported hearing the voices for the final time. 'We are pleased to have helped you. Goodbye', they said. She has since made a full recovery. See *Independent* 19 December 1997 and *Fortean Times* March 1998, no 108.

What these voices were, whether the information they provided was in some sense already known to the patient, remains open to speculation.

193  *Flesh of the Gods,* Peter T Furst (Ed), London 1972.

194 See Catherine Summers & Julian Vayne, *The Inner Space WorkBook*.

195 Telepathic experiences are also reported by many MDMA users see Bruce Eisner op cit.

196 See Lilly, *The Human Biocomputer*.

197 For an excellent example of 'supernatural' information arising in the mind during drug experience see Ann Shulgin's account in *PIHKAL*.

198 See Michael Harner, *The Way of the Shaman*, HarperCollins, 1990.

199 'The power of a particular experiment to replicate an effect also depends on how strong the effect is and how many observations are made...This is strikingly illustrated by a recent medical experiment designed to determine whether aspirin can prevent heart attacks. The study was discontinued in 1987 because it was already clear the answer was yes. After six years, the aspirin group had already suffered 45 percent fewer heart attacks than a control group that received only placebo medication, a result that would occur by chance less than one out of a million (The Steering Committee of the Physicians' Health Study Research Group, 1988)...The pertinent point here is that the study included over 22,000 subjects. If it were to be repeated with 3,000 subjects, a significant aspirin effect would be unlikely to emerge; the experiment would fail to replicate. Despite its undisputed reality and its practical importance, the aspirin effect is actually quite weak.'

See *Introduction to Psychology* Rita L.Atkinson, Richard C. Atklinson, Edward E.Smith, Daryl J.Bem, Harcourt Brace 1993.

Again the apparent simplicity of the experimental method can be muddied by introducing the placebo as a 'heart attack reduction drug'. Also findings such as this rest upon the idea that statistical analysis can provide us with ideas of significance based on our assumption that there are random but unlikely events in the universe. Thus we might analyse precognition by comparing a person's ability to predict a coin toss in relation to the number of heads and tails we should get 'by chance'. Naturally this leads to all kinds of questions, the most important being 'how do we know the value for chance?' With the advent of chaos mathematics, scientists are beginning to increasingly question whether there is any such thing as a 'random' event in the universe. Although we may not be able to predict a specific event with any certainty, science does now acknowledge that there can be complex, non-linear systems (such as fractals) which show self similarity at different scales (for example the way the branching system of veins in a leaf mimics in microcosm the overall shape of the whole tree). In practice this means that there are patterns, tendencies, and structures within events. These may be specifically unpredictable for a single event but, when viewed as a whole, they do show appreciable structure. The simplest way to think of this is to consider the weather. Each year Britain has a summer and winter but we can't really predict exactly when these seasons will happen. Equally we recognise clouds, and even certain classes of clouds, yet each cloud is different with an unpredictable shape and movement.

200 See Cynthia Giles model for how tarot reading might work in terms of quantum physics in *Tarot –The Complete Guide,* Hale, 1993. In modern occultism the understanding of magic in terms of current physics is a major element in the Chaos Magic schools, and is very significant in the work of occultists such as Pete Carroll.

201 Bruno la Tour, *Science in Action; How to follow Scientists and Engineers through Society*, Harvard University Press, 1987.

202 This tendency is roundly critiqued by Crowley in *Magick in Theory and Practice* and, in a more modern social context, by Monica Sjöö in *New Age and Armageddon; Towards a Feminist Vision of the Future*, The Women's Press, 1998.

203 See Starhawk, *Truth or Dare*, Harper and Row, 1990.

204 'According to primitive notions, all abnormal states - such as intoxication or madness – are caused by the entrance of a spirit into the person; such mental states, in other words, are regarded as forms of possession or inspiration.' See Frazer - *The Golden Bough* Vol 1.

205 Personally I don't see reification, i.e. treating metaphorical terms as though they were 'things', as a problem. As Jung points out in his commentary on *The Secret of the Golden Flower* (1957), when writing about personified archetypes in the context of religion. 'Many of the earlier gods developed from "persons" into personified ideas, and finally into abstract ideas. Activated unconscious content always appear at first as projections upon the outside world, but in the course of mental development they are gradually assimilated by consciousness and reshaped into conscious ideas that then forfeit their originally autonomous and personal character. As we know, some of the old gods have become, via astrology, nothing more than descriptive attributes (martial, jovial, saturnine, erotic, logical, lunatic, and so on)...We (Europeans) think we can congratulate ourselves on already having reached such a pinnacle of clarity; imagining that we have left all these phantasmal gods far behind. But what we have left behind are only verbal spectres, not the psychic facts that were responsible for the birth of the gods. We are still as much possessed by autonomous psychic

contents as if they were Olympians. Today they are called phobias, obsessions, and so forth; in a word, neurotic symptoms. The gods have become diseases; Zeus no longer rules Olympus but rather the solar plexus, and produces curious presentments for the doctor's consulting room, or disorders the brains of politicians and journalists who unwittingly let loose psychic epidemics on the world.'

206 To reiterate the relativity of this term, just as with 'drug' the definition of 'toxic' is a moot point. Sufficient doses of anything, water included, will irreparably damage the organism. Fortunately the omnivorous, scavenging, hunting and gathering strategies of human beings means that we can absorb quite a variety and range of different foods which, to various degrees stress the palate, digestive system or psyche.

207 This moment came as a wonderful epiphany. Having smoked whilst camped on a beach in southern France, I was delighted to 'become aware' that the cliff in front of me looked suddenly like a vast recumbent giant. The Mediterranean gave birth to the full moon and I genuinely wept to see how beautiful the world was (and is).

208 The narrative fiction of the self is described neatly by Carlos Casteneda as the 'point of assemblage' from where we build the universe. Part of the point of shamanic experience is to 'shake up' the individual so that he or she may decide to change their assemblage point – i.e. to transgress into the Other and learn.

209 'LSD and 5-HT Receptors', 1995 paper archived on the World Wide Web http://www.hyperreal.com

210 The notion of 'rulerships' in astrology is a form of the 'doctrine of signatures' or correspondence. See Crowley's *777*.

211 One model of LSD's effect has been advanced by John C. Lilly, 'In the analysis of the effects of LSD-25 on the human mind, a reasonable hypothesis states that the effect of these substances...is to introduce *white noise* (in the sense of a randomly varying energy containing no signals of itself )...One can thus "explain" the apparent speeding-up of subjective time; the enhancement of colors and detail in perceptions of the real world; the production of illusions; the freedom to make new programs; the appearance of visual projections onto mirror images of the real face and body; the projection and apparent depth in colored and in black-and-white photos; the projection of emotional expression onto other real persons; the synesthesia of music to visual projections; the feeling of "oneness with the universe"; apparent ESP effects; communications from "beings other than humans"; the lowered Cloze-analysis scores by outside

scorers; the clinical judgement of the outside observer of *dissociation psychosis, depersonalization, hallucination,* and *delusion* in regard to the subject; the apparent increase in muscular strength, and the dissolution and rebuilding of programs and metaprograms by self and by the outside therapist, etc.

The increase in *white noise* energy allows quick and random access to memory and lowers the threshold to unconscious memories (*expansion of consciousness*). In such noise one can project almost anything at almost any cognitive level in almost any allowable mode; one dramatic example is the conviction of some subjects of hearing-seeing-feeling God, when "way out". One projects one's expectations of God onto the white noise as if the noise were signals; one *hears the voice of God in the Noise*. With a bit of proper programming under the right conditions, with the right dose, at the right time, one can program almost anything into the noise within one's cognitive limits...

The noise introduced brings a certain amount of disorder with it, even as white noise in the physical world brings randomness. However, the LSD-25 noise randomizes signals only in a limited way; not enough to destroy all order, only enough to superimpose a small creative "jiggling" on program materials and metaprograms and their signals. The noisy component added to the usual signals in the circuits adds enough uncertainty to the meanings to make new interpretations more probable. If the noise becomes too intense, one might expect it to wipe out information and lead to unconsciousness (at very high levels, death).

The major operative principle seems to be that the human computer operates in such a way as to make signals out of the noise and thus to create information out of random energies where there was no signal.' See Lilly, John C. *The Human Biocomputer.*

212 The most easily obtained natural source of LSD type material is from the seeds of the Morning Glory plant. Again internet sites carry information on the use of this plant. Most companies who retail the seeds treat them with poisons to prevent their use as drugs.

213 Perhaps one might also compare LSD to the 19th Century notion of the god Pan, since as well as being awe-ful, and leading to heights of mystical revelation, acid can also be a trickster, a fun drug and one that can lead to laughter and capricious fun.

214 See Bruce Eisner op cit.

215 The harmful effects of Thalidomide were first made public in 1962.

216 See Jay Stevens, op cit.

217 In this paper Eisner also quotes one of the first people to create 'street acid' Bernard Roseman. 'Roseman, [who was] "…arrested for allegedly attempting to smuggle 62,000 doses of LSD." In Roseman's "LSD and the Age of the Mind", he recounts his experience of a "belt and braces" approach to pharmacology which resulted in less than pharmaceutically pure LSD. "LSD is a translucent crystal; this was a black mess. Thus, the first underground LSD was also the first impure batch, and its distribution may, somewhere, have incurred the first unfavourable consumer reaction." However Roseman's own description of taking his 'underground LSD' sounds like a perfectly wonderful trip "I had psychologically prepared myself for failure, so I just closed my eyes and lay back and listened to the wonderful sounds of Wagner. In my concentration, I failed to notice that the music was getting slowly louder and instead of just my ears hearing, all my senses seemed to encompass the sound., and instead of hearing the music - I was the music! Beautiful, soft colors emerged and exploded as climates of tone were achieved. An immediate understanding of the composer's intentions was revealed to me; I was being taken on a heavenly excursion into the world of pure sound and emotion. All at once, I sprang up with joy. I was in the state of LSD - my own LSD which I had made. I was deliriously happy and proud of my success.'

Once again, purity is often in the mind of the tripper.

218 'There are four possible isomers of LSD, but only the d-lysergic acid diethyl amide form is active. The other rotation forms - l-lysergic acid diethyl amide, d and l iso-lysergic acid diethyl amide (contrary to recent reports!) - are inactive. They have no pharmacological role, except possibly as a catalyst for some latent effect of LSD, or to block the action of LSD at the receptor site.' See Bruce Eisner, *High Times*, 1977.

219 One of the most common suggestions about the different effects of LSD is caused by the suggestion that street-acid contains strychnine. However as this information posted on the World Wide Web (at www.hyperreal.com) explains. . .The following text was written by Alexander T. Shulgin in response to the overwhelming misconception that strychnine is commonly found in street samples of LSD: 'The observation of strychnine as being present in any street drug, as a by-product, or a contaminant, or an impurity has never been documented. It is a natural plant product, as are the ergots which are used in the synthesis of LSD. But they come from totally unrelated plants; there has never been a report of strychnine and an ergot alkaloid co-existing in a single species. So if the two materials are

together in a drug sample, it could only be by the hand of man. I have personally looked at a large number of illicit street offerings and have never detected the presence of strychnine. The few times that I have indeed found it present, have been in legal exhibits where it usually occurred in admixture with brucine (also from the plant Strychnos nux-vomica) in criminal cases involving attempted or successful poisoning. The same argument applies to the myth that occasionally surfaces, that strychnine occurs in the white tufts of peyote. This is equally fraudulent — it has never been reported in that or any other cactus.

Furthermore, it should probably be spelled out that strychnine is not needed to bond LSD to blotter paper, nor is strychnine a breakdown product of LSD. These are probably the two most commonly repeated gross misconceptions.

The source of the "strychnine is commonly found in LSD" myth may be somewhat grounded in truth. For example, in "LSD: My Problem Child" Albert Hoffman cites a case in the late sixties of Strychnine being found in an "LSD" sample that was a white powder. However, what is commonly claimed is that strychnine is found in a significant percentage of LSD, specifically blotter LSD, which is not true. Shulgin's note that he has analyzed many samples of LSD and never found strychnine is backed up by published analyses done by PharmChem and the LA County Street Drug Analysis program, which likewise never found any strychnine.

This is intuitively backed up by the fact that a 5mm x 5mm "standard" square of blotter LSD only weights about 2mg and if the paper itself was made completely out of pure strychnine it is still on the very low end of Strychnine's threshold of activity.

Strychnine is not the cause of tracers, cramps, nausea, or amphetamine-like LSD-effects. It's possible that poorly synthesized LSD might have other ergot derivatives in it, which might contribute to the harsh body load that some get on taking LSD. Also, the very close chemical relatives 1-Methyl-LSD and 1-Acetyl-LSD (which breakdown into LSD in aqueous solution) might be present in some street samples and might contribute to the harsh body load. (Peter Stafford has claimed in his *Psychedelics Encyclopedia* that 1-Acetyl-LSD is supposedly "smoother" than d-LSD — thus "strychnine laced acid" may actually be pure d-LSD, while "pure LSD" may be 1-Acetyl-LSD or some substitute). And the chemicals iso-LSD and lumi-LSD which are breakdown products of LSD might contribute to the body loading on some trips, particularly via a hypothetical synergistic effect. Given this plethora of possible chemicals in street "LSD", its not needed to look to a chemical which has hardly ever been found in analyzed samples to explain variations in the strength and "cleanliness" of street acid. It's also possible that LSD itself simply causes adverse physical effects, particularly muscle cramping, in persons susceptible to it. The reported side effects of LSD (the nausea and apparent CNS stimulant effects) are commonly reported side effects of seritonergic drugs such as fluoxetine (Prozac) and buspirone (Buspar), and also are commonly reported (and typically more severe) with other psychedelics like Mescaline. Or it is quite likely that the "strychnine" reactions to LSD are entirely psychosomatic. Both Leary (*The Psychedelic Experience*) and Lilly (*Programming and Metaprogramming..., Center of the Cyclone*) have each observed this reaction in people who cannot handle the surge of emotion associated with a trip. Further advice would be to avoid methylxanthines (caffeine, theophylline in tea, etc) prior to dosing. Some have noted a possible synergistic effect between them and LSD causing, or contributing, to a harsh body load during a trip. And prior use of dramamine may alleviate the nausea sometimes associated with LSD, and other psychedelic drugs (although it may also effect the quality of the trip — Shulgin has noted in PIHKAL that he shuns the use of anti-nauseants in order to experience the effects of the psychedelic, both good and bad, with no possible interference).

In summary, it can't be said that we know specifically why sometimes acid feels "cleaner" than other times. However, based on the availability of plausible explanations, and the evidence of drug analysis, and general implausibility of the whole strychnine concept, we can conclude that it isn't due to any concentration of strychnine. Also, while it can't completely be ruled out, the presence of strychnine in LSD is so minimal that the majority of LSD users will never once come across it.

220 Abram Hoffer and Humphrey Osmond reported promising results in using LSD to treat alcoholism, schizophrenia and people with autism. See *New Hope for Alcoholics,* New York University Books, 1968. LSD has also recently been used, with apparently good results, see *The Treatment of childhood Schizophrenia Utilizing LSD and Psilocybin,* Gary Fisher, MAPS Volume 7, Number 3, Summer 1997.

221 See *Hygieia – A Woman's Herbal,* Jeannine Parvati, Freestone Collective, 1978.

222 Although I have read a number of accounts of fly agaric intoxication I have only had the opportunity to talk to one user who pressed the drug into what might be called 'shamanic service'. His account was that the drug was mildly psychedelic in that it produced a heightening state of awareness and

'strangeness' of mental state but without significant visuals. He also suggested that it produced a sense of being disembodied and walking, although not too difficult physically, felt like 'floating' (a number of accounts claim that the feet feel 'numb') across the ground. Accounts of fly agaric are quite disparate, suggesting that this is far from the most reliable psychedelic drug. Insofar as this is the case I agree with Terence McKenna in that Wasson's assumption that the ancient Indian Soma was identical with fly agaric, is doubtful.

223  See Henry Munn, *The Mushrooms of Language*, in *Hallucinogens and Shamanism* op cit.

224  See Terence McKenna, op cit.

225  Again there is an emphasis on graphic symbols or writing and therefore language in these hallucinations.

226  This suggestion is supported by Gerardo Reichel-Dolmatoff in *Drug-induced Optical Sensations and Their Relationship to Applied Art among some Colombian Indians,* see *Rainforest Shamans*.

227  This is the name given to the south American indigenous preparation which combines plants containing harmine, harmaline and DMT. The alkaloid harmine acts as a powerful MAO inhibitor causing the DMT component of the brew to become orally active.

228  Kundalini is the bio-sexual 'root energy' of the body which is raised in certain yogic practices and is vital to much of the tantrik tradition. This force may have some connection with a range of phenomena including spontaneous human combustion. See Larry E. Arnold, *Ablaze! Spontaneous Human Combustion*, M. Evans and Company, 1995. Sounds heard during the onset of a DMT trip are commonly reported as being like waterfalls, buzzing or ripping fabric.

229  See *Apparent Communication with Discarnate Entities Induced by Dimethyltryptamine (DMT),* by Peter Meyer (http://serendipity.magnet.ch/)

230  Although the content of pills, the 'substance', certainly has a bearing on their effect, there is just as much externalising of the effect of the drug experience onto the drug as with LSD use. For example it is commonly believed that some pills contain heroin, responsible for more mellow or perhaps bad and 'mongy' MDMA experiences. However, Matthew Collins writing on the known reports of ecstasy tests up until October 1993 says, 'heroin has never been found in tablets that contained MDMA; it had, however, been found in a handful of pills designed to simulate

Ecstasy that included other substances such as ephedrine.' See Matthew Collin (with John Godfrey) *Altered States* op cit.

231 Users should be conscious that no drugs effects are entirely predictable. A person who is suffering from serious depression or stress may well find the 'bursting the bubble' effect of MDMA (see Eisner op cit). In this situation emotional stress can turn the e-trip into a non-event or induce a general sense of melancholy. Although rare I have also come across one case in which an MDMA user was involved in an assault whilst on the drug. He subsequently has stopped using the drug since he was disturbed by how much he enjoyed and 'got into' fighting. This is unusual but should be born in mind when considering how the individual's history will affect the possible directions of their drug experience.

232 A German study showed that MDEA ('eve') produced an increase in responsiveness to emotions without anxiety. Sensitivity, perception, formal thought processes and memory were normal. MDEA has much the same effect as MDMA although the two drugs were not compared directly. See 'Psychological Effects of MDE in Normal Subjects', by Leo Hermle et al *Neuropsychopharmacology* 1993 8/2.

233 There seems to be very little research currently available into this area (since 'women's health and drug use' is, bizarrely, often considered as something of a 'minority' issue). The association between MDMA and heavy periods is paradoxical given the effects of amphetamine on menstruation, although research is complicated by the range of substances that are sold in 'pills'. For research on pregnant animal studies see Nicholas Saunders *Ecstasy and the Dance Culture* op cit.

234 See *Euphoria* archives at www.hyperreal.com

235 A major neurotransmitter. Speed may also have effects on the dopamine.

236 Andrew Tyler *Street Drugs* op cit.

237 See Sigmund Freud *The Cocaine Papers,* Dunquin Press, 1963.

238 Robert Sabbag op cit..

239 The Tantrik 'goddess' or representation of the primal feminine or 'Other', identical with Crowley's goddess Babalon.

240 (Mahapurush Ram Giri) in *Drugs and Sexuality* David Solomon and George Andrews (Eds).

241 Medical use of opiates usually involves diamorphine which is between three and four times more potent than morphine.

242 Thomas De Quincey, *The Pleasures and Pains of Opium*, Penguin 1995.

243 Reported in *New Scientist*, 'Prisoners of Pleasure' by David Concar and Rosie Mestel, October 1994.

244 See Eric Simon, *Substance Abuse: A Comprehensive Textbook*, William & Wilkins, Baltimore 1992.

245 See *Drugs and Pharmacology for Nurses*, S.J.Hopkins, Churchill Livingstone, 1995. Although hallucinations are a common part of the ketamine experience. Texts which focus on the use of ketamine as an anaesthetic for other animals obviously miss this phenomena. For instance 'In studies involving 14 species of subhuman primates…Recovery is generally smooth and uneventful. The duration is dose related.' From archives at www.hyperreal.com. Of course if we could ask the primates what they thought about the drug they might report matters quite differently.

246 See Terence McKenna, op cit.

247 The magician Austin Osman Spare used his tobacco addiction as a way of casting spells. He would repress his magical desire (what he referred to as a 'sigil') into the unconscious by focusing his attention on giving up smoking. His aim was to deliberately forget his sigil so that it could grow to manifestation, uninterrupted by the conscious attention of his mind.

248 See J.Ott *The Cacahuatl Eater: Ruminations of an Unabashed Chocolate Eater*, Natural Products Co., 1985.

249 See Terence McKenna, op cit.

250 Distributed by promoters of the drug and available via www.hyperreal.com

251 The following account is from Gracie and Zarkov and is drawn from the archives at www.hyperreal.com. It recounts the effect of an accidental high dose 2-CB experiment. The experimenters' own thoughts on the role of 2-CB as a somatic hallucinogen which targets the 'reptile brain' are included.

'The peak effects could be roughly categorized under visual, emotional and somatic modes. However, these three modes were out of synch: the visual disturbances did not correlate to the emotional feelings, nor either of the former to somatic sensations. By concentrating attention on one of the modes, all three would moderate. This was especially noted by Zarkov, who was able to deal with the peak effect without losing it by focusing attention on a particular effect. For example, the overwhelming feeling of terror at the peak was unlike a DMT, LSD or Psilocybian mushroom trip where there is an apparent causal or precipitating incident, vision, encounter or meaningful train of thought (e.g. something is threatening one, or one encounters personal demons, etc.) 2CB terror had no discernible "cause". Upon self-reflection, no cause could be found. "Why am I terrorized?" was a question with no answer. This self-reflection produced a significant decrease in the feeling of terror. Zarkov remarked, "It was as if 2CB was a specific chemical agent exciting a "terror circuit" in your brain to overload with no object, no insight and no cause.'

For 30 minutes to 1 hour, 30 minutes we felt increasing nausea, GI cramps, the kind of symptoms Gracie associates with extreme anxiety, fear or anger. Chills and shakes appeared physiological rather then psychosomatic, since they went away with the hot bath. The somatic sensations were quite overwhelming, and like the terror described above, had no discernible cause except (speculating) limbic hyperarousal. Animal arousal continued throughout the trip, accompanied by tactile sensitivity, skin flushing and erectile tissue engorgement. However, neither of us found those effects erotic. Any level of activity — bathing, removing contact lenses, crawling around — reduced somatic effects. There was no appetite suppression, unlike methoxylated amphetamines.

Our present model for understanding this is based on the Leary-Wilson 8 circuits model, which seems to place such raging neurosomatic surges into the lowest (biosurvival) circuit. Metaphorically and phylogenetically speaking, it represents the lizard component of your bodymind — the limbic system which controls and produces 'fight, flight, feed or fuck' behaviour (the 4 Fs). Think of an aroused alligator, thrashing snake or cranked-up dinosaur: powerful and active, but with a surging chemical or emotional drive more primitive and older than our monkey ways of behaving. Interestingly, the emotional effects were clearly related to some of the somatic effects in that concentrating on emotions relieved the body reactions. For example, Gracie found that the gastrointestinal cramps, nausea and unpleasant (to put it mildly!) feelings melted away when she focused on the emotional pain, rage, fear or desire — crying, sobbing, wailing, howling or clinging all helped to alleviate the discomfort. As described above, focusing on one component of the trip made the others fade away. Physical activity would also relieve the physical and emotional distress, e.g. dancing, thrashing, crawling around.

After the Peak

Gracie remarked that the trip was like a Puccini opera — lots of emotional manipulation but lacking in depth. We returned to our trip room and played heavy metal rock (Blue Cheer) which helped greatly to restore our equilibrium. Gracie danced, growled, crawled around and raved about "barbarian hordes from the Id" (not a rock band). From then on, we both improved markedly, became euphoric and stayed aroused. The unpleasant body symptoms slowly faded.'

252 Researches into the effects of ibogaine include the Pharmacology and Toxicology Department of Albany Medical College, headed by Dr. Stanley D. Glick. also Nathan S. Kline Institute for Psychiatric Research, a facility of the New York State Office of Mental Health affiliated with NYU Medical Centre, and the City University of New York Medical School.

253 See Glick, 'Effects of Ibogaine on Acute Signs of Morphine Withdrawal in Rats: Independence from Tremor', *Neuro-pharmacology*, Vol. 31, No. 5, p. 497-500, 1992.

254 Andrew Tyler op cit.

255 See *The Iboganie story - Report on the Staten Island Project,* Paul de Rienzo, Dana Beal & members of the project, in print and also at http://www.cures-not-wars.org/ibogaine/iboga.html.

256 And, 'From the reports of human heroin addicts who have taken ibogaine, it appears that several features of the ibogaine experience are important in interrupting addiction. Thus, Dutch addicts who used ibogaine described the experience as having a dream with full consciousness, together with anxiety and the recall of memories. After this experience, the addicts did not feel compelled to use heroin. While these insights are intriguing, they are at present without heuristic value. Further studies are required to determine the importance of such experiences in the treatment of drug abuse. In conclusion, the claimed "anti-addictive" properties of ibogaine require rigorous validation in humans, after careful assessment of its neurotoxic potential. It remains to be established if an ibogaine metabolite,

producing less side effects, could be of therapeutic value.' See Lotsof, H.S., *Ibogaine in the treatment of chemical dependency disorders: clinical perspectives,* MAPS, 1995, 5: 16-27. and Kaplan, C.D., Ketzer, E., de Jong, J. and de Vries, M., 'Reaching a state of wellness: Multistage explorations in social neuroscience.' *Social Neuroscience Bulletin,* 1993, 6: 6-7.

257 As mentioned earlier I feel there is no doubt that animal testing can and does provide useful information about drugs. However this does not necessarily mean that it is a)morally okay or b)that it shows the most important actions of the drug. This is especially important with drugs that have significant psychological effects.

258 Anyone who wants to experiment with new drugs, particularly the more exotic plants and materials that can be used to change consciousness is well advised to spend a few days surfing the internet to get a good sample of information. There are a number of excellent books that cover this area, including *Plants of the Gods* (op cit.) and *Legal Highs,* Adam Gottlieb, 20th Century Alchemist, 1992.

259 See *The Forbidden Game – A Social History of Drugs,* Brian Inglis, Coronet 1977.

260 I would urge all readers who feel that they would like to engage with the political aspects of drug legislation to contact Transform which is a UK anti-prohibitionist movement at http://www.transform-drugs.org.uk/

261 Matthew Collin (with John Godfrey) op cit.

262 Simon Reynolds in *The Wire,* 1992

263 Altered States op cit.

264 See *The Doors of Perception/Heaven and Hell,* Harper, 1954.

265 See *She Comes in Colors* interview with Timothy Leary in *Playboy* magazine September 1966.

266 Richard Alpert (Ram Dass) 'LSD and Sexuality' published in *The Psychedelic Review* 1969.

267 Indeed 'art' in many ways is itself a 'liminal material' (try asking yourself the simple question 'what is art?'). Certain art forms are directly in touch with what Eliade calls the 'shamanic complex'. For instance, in talking about

crop circles as art one commentator writes; 'While mostly outside the parameters of conventional art practice, this type of folk art embraces that rich vein of mythology occupied by the trickster. Far from being a cynic or a sceptic, the trickster, from shamanic cultures to our own, has punctuated history with lies and deceptions. The resulting collision of genuine and fake, artifice and reality, has created a paradoxical twilight reality that is the arena of strange phenomena. Artists have found and populated this arena for decades, perhaps even centuries, regularly producing representations which, at their best, are visionary works of art." Rob Dickinson, *Fortean Times*, 106 1997.

268 The surrealist movement was far from noted in its use of drugs to gain altered states, but one of the movement's seminal texts, *The Lay of Maldoror* (by Comte de Lautréamont) may well have been inspired, in part, by visions obtained under the influence of deadly nightshade. Atropine, a powerful toxin found in nightshade, is a central nervous stimulant. Depending on dosage effects can range from talkativeness and physical agitation, through excitement and 'delirium', to paralysis and collapse. Lautréament was found dead in Paris aged only twenty-four, possibly due to deadly nightshade poisoning.

269 See Oliver Sacks, *Seeing Voices,* University of California Press, 1989.

270 The distinction between logical and emotional thought can also be deconstructed from within the discourse of science, see Antonio Damasio's *Descartes' Error* op cit.

271 See J.Bruner, *Acts of Meaning*, Harvard University Press, 1990.

272 See Albert Hofmann, *LSD My Problem Child*.

# Bibliography

Arnold, Larry E. *Ablaze! Spontaneous Human Combustion* M.Evans and Company 1995

Baron-Cohen, Dr Simon & Bolton, Dr Patrick *Autism - the Facts* OUP 1993

Berman, David (Editor) *Modern Philosophy of the Mind* Everyman 1995

Bey, Hakim *The Temporary Autonomous Zone, Ontological Anarchy, Poetic Terrorism* Autonomedia 1991

Blakemore, Colin *The Mind Machine* Penguin 1994

Bruner, J. *Acts of Meaning* Harvard University Press 1990

Bunney, Sarah (ed.) *The Illustrated Book of Herbs* Octopus 1987

Carroll, Pete *Liber Null & Psychonaut* Weiser 1987

Carroll, Peter J, *Psybermagick* Chaos International & Asafoetida 1995.

Cocteau, Jean *Opium* Peter Owen 1968

Collins, Jeff & Mayblin, Bill (Illustrator) *Derrida for Beginners* Icon Books 1997

Crowley, Aleister *777 & Other Qabalistic Writings* Weiser 1986

Crowley, Aleister *Magick In Theory and Practice* Routledge and Kegan Paul 1983

Crowley, Aleister *The Book of Thoth* Wesier 1980

Csikszentmihalyi, Mihaly *Creativity : Flow and the Psychology of Discovery and Invention* HarperCollins 1996

Culling, Louis T *A Manual of Sex Magick* Llewellyn 1971.

Culling, Louis T. *The Complete Magick Curriculum of the Secret Order G.B.G.* Llewellyn 1969

Damasio, Antonio R. *Descartes' Error* Picador 1996

De Quincey, Thomas *The Pleasures and Pains of Opium* Penguin 1995

Dennett, Daniel *Consciousness Explained* Penguin 1991.

Diamond, Jared *The Rise and Fall of the Third Chimpanzee* Vintage 1991

Duerr, Hans Peter *Dreamtime: concerning the boundary between wilderness and civilization* Basil Blackwell 1985.

Edelman, Gerald *Bright Air, Brilliant Fire* HarperCollin 1992

Edwards, Betty *Drawing on the Left Hand Side of the Brain* Fontana 1979

Eisner, Bruce *Ecstasy: The MDMA Story* Ronin Publishing 1989.

Eliade , Mircea *Shamanism: Archaic Techniques of Ecstasy* Bollingen 2004

Fortune, Dion *Psychic Self-Defence* Aquarian 1967

Foucault, Michel. *Madness and Civilisation* Random House 1965

Foucault, Michel. *The Order of Things* Tavistock 1970

Frazer, J. *The Golden Bough: A Study in Magic and Religion: A New Abridgement from the Second and Third Editions* Oxford World's Classics 1998

Freud, Sigmund *The Cocaine Papers* Dunquin Press 1963

Furst, Peter T (Editor) *Flesh of the Gods* London 1972

Geschwind, N. & Galaburda, A.M *Cerebral Lateralization* Bradford 1987.

Giles, Cynthia *Tarot –The Complete Guide* Hale 1993

Gladstone, Ralph *Marijuana Papers* 1972

Goldman, Albert *Disco* Hawthorn Books 1978

Gottlieb, Adam *Legal Highs* 20th Century Alchemist 1992

Grant, Kenneth *Aleister Crowley and the Hidden God* Muller 1973

Grinspoon, Lester *Marihuana Reconsidered* Harvard University Press 1971

Gross, Richard D *Psychology* Hodder & Stoughton 1992

Harding, Elizabeth U. *Kali, The Black Goddess of Dakshineswar* Nicholas-Hays 1993

Harner, Michael (Editor) *Hallucinogens and Shamanism* Oxford University Press 1973

Hine, Phil *Walking Between the Worlds – techniques of modern shamanism* Pagan News Publications 1989

Hoffer, Abram & Osmond, Humphrey *New Hope for Alcoholics* New York University Books 1968

Hofmann, Albert & Schultes, Richard Evans *Plants of the Gods* Healing Arts Press 1992.

Hofmann, Albert *LSD My Problem Child* McGraw-Hill 1980

Hopkins, S.J. *Drugs and Pharmacology for Nurses* Churchill Livingstone 1995

Howard, Judy *The Bach Flower Remedies Step by Step* C.W.Daniel, 1990.

Humphrey Nicholas, *A History of the Mind* Vintage 1993

Husserl, Edmund *Ideas* Collier 1962

Huxley, Aldous *The Doors of Perception/Heaven and Hell* Harper 1954

Inglis, Brian *The Forbidden Game – A Social History of Drugs* Coronet 1977

Jung, C.G. (Editor) & Wilhelm, Richard (Translator) *The Secret of the Golden Flower : Chinese Book of Life* Arkana 1988

Koestler, Arthur *The Ghost in the Machine* Hutchinson 1967

la Tour, Bruno *Science in Action; How to follow Scientists and Engineers through Society* Harvard University Press 1987.

LaChapelle, Dollores *Sacred Land, Sacred Sex, Rapture of The Deep* Finn Hill Arts 1988.

Laing, RD & Esterson, A. *Sanity Madness and the Family* Basic Books 1964

Leary, Timothy *The Politics of Ecstasy* Ronin Publishing, 1997

Lickey, Marvin and Gordon, Barbara *Drugs for Mental Illness* W.H.Freeman and Company 1983.

Lilly,John C. *The Human Biocomputer* Abacus 1967

Lventhal, H. *In the Shadow of the Enlightenment* New York University Press 1976

Maslow, Abraham H. *Motivation and Personality* Harper and Row 1970

Maslow, Abraham H. *Towards a Psychology of Being* Harper & Row 1968

Mathers, S. L. MacGregor (Editor) *The Goetia the Lesser Key of Solomon the King* Weiser Books 1995

McKenna, Terence *Food of the Gods* Rider 1992

Michel Foucault *Madness and Civilisation* Random House 1965

Mrsich W., *Erfahrungen mit Hexen und Hexensalbe* Germany 1957

Ott J., *The Cacahuatl Eater: Ruminations of an Unabashed Chocolate Eater* Natural Products Co. 1985

Paracelsus, Nicholas Goodrick-Clarke (Editor) *Essential Readings* North Atlantic Books 1999

Parvati, Jeannine *Hygieia – A Woman's Herbal* Freestone Collective 1978

Peter T (Editor) *Flesh of the Gods: The Ritual Use of Hallucinogens* Waveland Press 1990

Redgrove, Peter *The Black Goddess and the Sixth Sense* Paladin 1987

Regardie, Israel *The Golden Dawn* Llewellyn 1989

Reichel-Dolmatoff, Gerardo *Rainforest Shamans* Green Books 1997

Roney-Dougal, Serena *Where Science and Magic Meet* Element 1991

Russell, Jeffrey B. *A History of Witchcraft: Sorcerers, Heretics, and Pagans* Thames & Hudson 1982

Sabbag, Robert *Snowblind* Pan Books 1979

Sacks, Oliver *Seeing Voices* University of California Press 1989

Sacks, Oliver *The Man Who Mistook his Wife for a Hat* HarperCollins 1990

Saunders, Nicholas *Ecstasy and the Dance Culture* Nicholas Saunder 1995

Schueler, Gerald J. *Enochian Magic* Llewellyn 1988

Shulgin, Ann & Alexander *TIHKAL: The Continuation* Transform Press 1997

Shulgin, Ann and Alexander *PIHKAL: A Chemical Love Story* Transform Press 1991

Silverberg, R. *Drug Themes in Science Fiction* US Government National Institute of Drug Abuse 1973

Simeon, Abraham ben *The book of the sacred magic of Abra-Melin the Mage: As delivered by Abraham the Jew unto his son Lamech, A.D. 1458* J.M. Watkins 1900

Simon, Eric *Substance Abuse: A Comprehensive Textbook* William & Wilkins, Baltimore 1992

Sjöö, Monica *New Age and Armageddon; Towards a Feminist Vision of the Future* The Women's Press 1998

Solomon, David and Andrews, George (Editors) *Drugs and Sexuality* Panther Books 1973

Starhawk *Truth or Dare* Harper and Row 1990

Stevens, Jay *Storming Heaven; LSD and the American Dream* Paladin 1989

Summers, Catherine & Vayne, Julian *Seeds of Magick* W.Foulsham 1990

Summers, Catherine & Vayne, Julian *The Inner Space WorkBook* Capall Bann 1994

Summers, Montague (Editor) *The Malleus Maleficarum of Kramer and Sprenger* Dover Publications 1971

Taylor, Timothy *The Prehistory of Sex* Fourth Estate 1996

Tsuang, Ming T *Schizophrenia The Facts* OUP 1982

Tyler, Andrew *Street Drugs* Hodder & Stoughton 1995

Wasson, Robert Gordon *Soma: Divine Mushroom of Immortality* Harcourt 1972

Watts, Alan *The Joyous Cosmology* Jonathan Cape Ltd 1974

Winnicott, D.W *Playing and Reality* Routledge 1971

Winnicott, D.W. *Playing and Reality* Routledge, 1971

Zimmer, Lynn & Morgan, John P. *Marijuana Myths Marijuana Facts* Lindesmith Centre 1997

Zoja, Luigi *Drugs, Addiction and Initiation* Daimon 2000

# Index

## Symbols

2-CB   13, 149, 213, 214, 253, 266

## A

addiction   121, 143, 144, 202, 206, 207, 208, 215, 216, 222, 268
AI   115, 116, 117. *See also* See artificial intelligence
Alcohol   34, 210, 212
alcohol   13, 20, 27, 30, 42, 58, 128, 129, 147, 149, 179, 199, 203, 212, 215, 219, 220, 243, 245
Alpert   228
Amphetamine   25, 198
amphetamine   32, 33, 104, 109, 194, 198, 199, 202, 214, 219, 220, 249, 262, 265
amphetamines   104, 165, 200, 202, 238, 267
Apuleius   161
Artaud   37, 240
Artificial intelligence   115. *See also* See AI
Aspergers syndrome   87, 90
astrology   181, 241, 258, 259
Atavistic Resurgence   162
autism   86, 87, 88, 89, 90, 91, 93, 94, 96, 98, 99, 100, 101, 102, 103, 104, 106, 107, 108, 109, 110, 111, 112, 113, 127, 128, 134, 138, 246, 249, 251, 263
autopoiesis   62, 208
autopoietic   62, 63, 64, 65, 129, 233. *See also* See autopoiesis
ayahuasca   82, 151, 157, 166, 189, 192, 193

## B

Babalon'   61
Bataille   137, 243
Blackmore   152
Bruno   150, 241, 258
Buckmaster Fullers   60

## C

cannabis   14, 36, 40, 44, 48, 58, 104, 128, 178, 179, 180, 205, 212, 221, 243
Carroll   84, 125, 237, 258
catatonia   92
cerebral dominance   77, 78, 90. *See also* See lateralisation
chi   49
Christ   57, 62
Christian   49, 129, 132, 193, 251
coagula   14, 75, 100, 181
coca   46, 200
cocaine   20, 26, 42, 47, 59, 81, 119, 123, 198, 200, 201, 202, 203, 206, 208, 212, 215, 219
Collin   223, 225, 265, 269
Collins   59, 264
commissurotomy   86
computer   26, 107, 115, 116, 117, 132, 134, 135, 218, 249, 255, 260
Conan Doyle   59
Crowley   34, 61, 159, 231, 237, 239, 244, 247, 252, 255, 258, 259, 265

## D

Damasio   121, 251, 270
Datura   192, 247
datura   48, 93, 126, 128, 137, 142, 157, 235, 252
Dennett   101, 114, 120, 245, 249
Derrida   7, 23, 27, 140, 179, 233

277

Derridian 98, 231, 241. *See also* See Derrida
Desana 74, 75, 245
Descarte 81, 83, 114
Devil 49, 51
dexedrine 104, 194
Divination 168
DMT 59, 82, 83, 151, 152, 174, 189, 190, 191, 192, 206, 238, 246, 248, 253, 264, 267
DNA 161
Dolmatoff 75, 245, 264
dopamine 71, 73, 85, 103, 104, 106, 107, 108, 110, 111, 201, 203, 205, 206, 249, 265
D'Quicy 59
dualism 18, 68, 72, 114, 164
Duerr 53, 55, 160, 161, 242, 254, 256

## E

Ecstasy 193, 194, 195, 196, 214, 223, 240, 243, 251, 265. *See also* See MDMA
Edelman 116, 250
Eisner 182, 183, 194, 243, 250, 257, 260, 261, 265
Eleusis 30, 31
Eliade 45, 61, 241, 269
Entheogen 165
ESP 169, 259. *See also* See telepathy
ethnopharmacology 178

## F

Fenfluramine 104, 106
Fortean Times 165, 250, 254, 256, 270
Fortune 41, 240
Freud 63, 110, 155, 201, 207, 251, 265

## G

Gazzanigna 78
gender 42, 47, 139, 153, 251
Godfrey 223, 265, 269
Goldman 56, 242

## H

hallucination 89, 107, 126, 134, 163, 191, 195, 260
hallucinations 33, 36, 72, 80, 83, 91, 92, 95, 96, 97, 98, 103, 104, 106, 109, 110, 111, 112, 113, 151, 186, 190, 192, 208, 209, 252, 264, 266
hallucinogens 20, 28, 29, 85, 164, 186, 187, 252
harmaline 82, 264
harmine 82, 264
Harner 232, 240, 252, 257
Hermetic 93, 138, 159
Heroin 205, 206, 250
heroin 20, 42, 118, 120, 204, 205, 206, 264, 268
Hersch 95
HGA. *See* See Holy Guardian Angel
Hofmann 17, 32, 47, 60, 175, 176, 183, 184, 188, 234, 238, 270
Huxley 28, 29, 31, 224, 225, 227, 233

## I

Iain M.Banks 116
ibogaine 215, 216, 217, 268
Inglis 221, 269
interactionalism 114

## J

Jaynes 95

## K

kalas 145, 146, 147, 148

Kasparov 116
Ketamine 33, 208, 209
khat 217
Koestler 140, 252

## L

Lacan 136, 251
lateralisation 73, 74, 77, 79, 85, 249
Leadbeater 159
Leary 28, 29, 40, 117, 222, 225, 226, 227, 228, 240, 263, 267, 269
Lewin 33, 35
Lewis 150
Lilly 117, 169, 255, 257, 259, 260, 263
liminal 13, 14, 16, 19, 20, 29, 39, 53, 55, 57, 64, 79, 91, 128, 144, 147, 153, 154, 155, 163, 171, 173, 231, 234, 237, 242, 248, 269
Lipton 111
LSD 17, 27, 28, 29, 30, 31, 32, 37, 42, 59, 60, 80, 85, 104, 106, 111, 117, 122, 123, 124, 141, 158, 163, 169, 171, 175, 176, 177, 180, 181, 182, 183, 184, 185, 186, 188, 192, 197, 201, 203, 205, 206, 209, 212, 219, 221, 225, 227, 228, 234, 246, 248, 249, 250, 259, 260, 261, 262, 263, 264, 267, 269, 270
LSD-25 175, 259. See also See LSD

## M

magic 13, 14, 19, 32, 36, 38, 42, 45, 47, 122, 153, 154, 162, 166, 171, 173, 187, 231, 232, 234, 237, 240, 252, 254, 255, 256, 258

magician 47, 61, 63, 138, 150, 153, 159, 172, 173, 184, 219, 224, 237, 241, 255, 266
MAO inhibitors 82, 189, 219, 245. See also See MAOI
Marijuana 124, 243, 251. See also See Cannabis
Maslow 138, 244
materialist 107, 114, 115, 116, 117, 119, 127, 151, 156, 158, 173, 234
McGinn 114
McKenna 28, 30, 42, 156, 180, 187, 189, 190, 191, 246, 251, 253, 264, 266
MDMA 13, 25, 26, 28, 33, 42, 43, 111, 112, 119, 120, 123, 149, 169, 186, 193, 194, 195, 196, 197, 198, 203, 206, 212, 213, 214, 218, 219, 225, 241, 243, 246, 252, 257, 264, 265
meditation 36, 92, 122, 138, 185, 194, 195, 203, 222
melatonin 82, 83, 85
Mescaline 16, 28, 263
methylamphetamine 198
Moliere 102
Monmouth 164
morphine 121, 122, 148, 197, 204, 207, 216, 266
Munn 187, 264
mushrooms 30, 42, 44, 49, 147, 186, 187, 188, 189, 192, 201, 217, 218
mystery 13, 14, 104, 150

## N

Neitzche 37, 137
Newsome 204
Nietzsche 28, 240, 243
norepinephrine 121, 199, 201, 245

## O

occultism 12, 13, 14, 19, 61, 84, 85, 93, 120, 138, 159, 245, 254, 258
Opiates 205, 206, 207. *See also* See opium
Opium 32, 34, 59, 203, 205, 256, 266
opium 26, 32, 44, 102, 179, 204, 205, 206, 207, 208, 218, 256
Ornstein 75
Oswley 40
Ott 211, 266
Owsley 183

## P

Pagan 12, 153, 254
paradoxical effect 105, 109, 194, 202
PCP 183
peaking 185
Peyote 33
peyote 30, 128, 137, 148, 187, 188, 239, 262
phenylalkylamines 42
Piaget 127
placebo 25, 121, 122, 123, 124, 126, 142, 148, 177, 250, 257
Prozac 25, 105, 109, 112, 122, 144, 263
psilocybin 40, 111, 183, 184, 186, 188, 189, 192
psychedelic 15, 30, 33, 35, 36, 40, 44, 45, 48, 59, 63, 82, 85, 89, 91, 93, 117, 147, 148, 157, 165, 175, 179, 180, 181, 183, 186, 187, 189, 190, 191, 196, 197, 198, 201, 203, 205, 209, 211, 214, 216, 217, 225, 238, 245, 246, 248, 263

psychonauts 224

## Q

Qabalah 34, 159
Qabalistic 33, 34, 47, 239, 255. *See also* See Qabalah

## R

Redgrove 125, 251, 253
reverse tolerance 124
Reynolds 223, 269
Ritalin 108, 109, 198
ritual 15, 29, 32, 37, 45, 46, 58, 117, 122, 138, 142, 143, 148, 149, 153, 154, 182, 185, 186, 187, 210, 216, 229, 252, 254
Robert Sabbag 59, 202, 243, 265
Roney-Dougal 167, 237, 246, 250
Roosevelt 222

## S

Sacks 125, 165, 231, 246, 270
Salvia divinorum 165, 245
Satan 56, 68. *See also* See Devil
Saunders 70, 123, 194, 195, 251, 265
Saussure 23
Schizophrenia 92, 112, 127, 240, 246, 247, 248, 263
schizophrenia 37, 86, 91, 92, 93, 94, 96, 98, 99, 100, 101, 102, 103, 104, 105, 106, 107, 108, 109, 110, 111, 112, 113, 128, 134, 137, 138, 139, 247, 248, 249, 254, 263
schizophrenic 92, 93, 94, 96, 98, 104, 107, 110, 111, 112, 113, 120, 128, 135, 137, 140, 155, 167, 254
serotonin 25, 26, 71, 73, 82, 85, 101, 102, 103, 104, 105, 106, 107, 108, 111,

120, 121, 155, 180, 196, 205, 206, 245, 248, 249
shaman' 45, 46, 164. *See also* See Shamanic
shamanic 35, 38, 45, 46, 48, 49, 50, 52, 62, 75, 122, 130, 137, 138, 142, 147, 150, 151, 155, 156, 157, 158, 160, 161, 162, 171, 172, 173, 176, 181, 184, 193, 210, 227, 233, 240, 252, 254, 259, 263, 269. *See also* See Shaman
Sharon 168
Shulgin 15, 16, 61, 124, 178, 233, 237, 241, 243, 251, 256, 257, 261, 262, 263
skunk 141. *See also* See Cannabis
solve 14, 75, 100, 181
Spare 162, 253, 255, 266
Speed 198, 265. *See also* See amphetamine
Steven 7, 102, 117

# T

tantric. *See* See tantra
Tantrik 136, 145, 148, 253, 265
tao 16
Tarot 4
Taylor 100, 248
tea 129, 210, 263
telepathic 88, 166, 167, 168, 249
telepathy 89, 94, 152, 160, 168, 171, 256
Theophile Gautier 59
Thornapple 83. *See also* See Datura
Thugee 58, 243
tobacco 20, 42, 179, 210, 211, 266
transgression 16, 17, 18, 19, 32, 38, 49, 53, 65, 90, 118, 129, 130, 132, 136, 137, 138, 139, 140, 141, 145, 148, 149, 162, 172, 181,

186, 208, 222, 224, 229, 231, 233, 243, 251, 253
tryptamine 28, 151, 186
Tsuang 103, 104, 246, 247
Tyler 216, 251, 265, 268

# U

UFO 152

# V

Valdez 168
Vama Marg 136
Viagra 26
Voygotsky 63

# W

War on Drugs 222, 230
Wasson 28, 29, 156, 189, 241, 264
Watts 18, 237
Wicca 154. *See also* See Wiccan
Wiccan 98, 153
Wilbert 156
Winnicott 233, 237, 247
witch 47, 49, 50, 51, 52, 53, 54, 55, 56, 57, 153, 157, 161, 162, 163, 173, 242
witchcraft 49, 51, 52, 54, 57, 241, 242. *See also* See Witch

# X

XTC 225. *See also* See MDMA

# Y

yang 105
yin 105, 244
yoga 92, 203, 204

# Z

Zen 92, 194, 195, 205, 209
Zoja 144
zone of proximal development 64, 128

# Mandrake

## Now That's What I Call Chaos Magick
Greg Humphries & Julian Vayne (with foreword by Dave Lee)
£12.99 ISBN 1869928741 188pp

'we cannot recommend this book to anybody who is frightened of magic, of self-discovery or of adventure; to anybody who wants ritual experiences that are absolutely risk-free and have a guaranteed result; to anybody whose concept of ceremony depends on the provision of scripts for all participants, carefully typed out and enclosed in polythene wrappers; to anybody who believes that magical practices should follow set traditions, . . .; to anybody who believes that human beings are firmly subordinated to deities and must do their will; and to anybody whose favourite words of condemnation for others are 'irresponsible' or 'self-indulgent'. Above all, I cannot recommend it to anybody without a sense of humour. Anybody else should love it: it provides an experience of ritual that is energetic, fresh, investigative, exciting and fun, in a completely individual way.'
— Ronald Hutton.

## Chaotopia!: Sorcery and Ecstasy in the 5th Aeon
by Dave Lee
£12.99, ISBN 1869928881, 208pp

'Once one is fairly competent at practical sorcery, there is little of importance that remains to be said or read about the subject; the magician at this point tends to emphasize inner development in his work. It seems to me that Chaos Magic itself has reached this point; the basic ideas needed for anyone to construct his or her own system of sorcery and to hone their skills are already covered by the available books. What has been lacking so far, is a Chaos magical approach to the investigation of the ecstatic states that underlie magical gnosis. This book, rather than trying to provide yet another slightly different flavour of Chaos technique, takes as its starting point the relationship between ecstasy and magic; between Chaos Magic and Chaos Mysticism, if you like.' extract from page 8

'A highly intelligent book by a leading Chaos Magician which will broaden and deepen Chaoist debate, theory and practice.'
- Peter J. Carroll

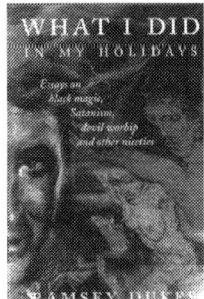
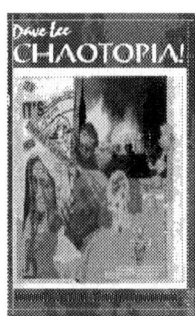
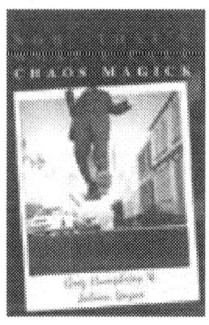
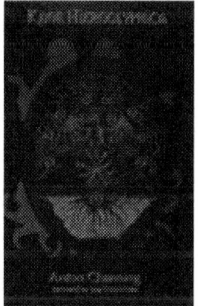

## What I did On My Holidays - Essays on Black Magic, Satanism and Devil Worship
by Ramsey Dukes
£18/$35, ISBN 1869928520, 420pp.

Is it ok for a national government to negotiate with terrorists? Should we be prepared to make a pact with the demon Terrorism - or should we remain forever sworn to the demon No Compromise? Many old and new demons lurk on these pages: black magic, sexism, elitism, satanism, publishers, prejudice, suicide, liberalism, violence, slime, old age, bitterness, war and the New Age.

Ramsey Dukes, patron saint of Chaos Magick, was incarnate around 1970 - occupying the body of a young Cambridge maths scholar with a long standing interest in magic, alchemy, Aleister Crowley and the occult.

## Kaos Hieroglyphica Alchemy for the New Aeon
By Anton Channing
£20/$35 ISBN 1869928830 200pp, special hardback, illustrated

In the year 1564, Dr John Dee published his work, Monas Hieroglyphica. Its central symbol represented the unity which was the gnosis of the monotheistic aeon.

Now over four hundred years later, Anton Channing has published his long awaited debut work Kaos Hieroglyphica, within which he expounds a new symbol, the Kaos Hieroglyph. This symbol represents the plurality and freedom of the New Aeon. This work of magical alchemy draws on such diverse material as Thelema, the Chaos Current, the Maat Current, Timothy Leary, Witchcraft, Paganism, the Hermetic Tradition, Taoism, Shamanism and the author's own Pineal Gland.

The Kaos Hieroglyphica offers the reader interpretations of Hermetic symbolism in a way that is both insightful and relevant to New Aeon Magic.

## Visual Magick: A Manual of Freestyle Shamanism
By Jan Fries
£10.99/$20. ISBN 1869928-571, 196pp

A new edition of the highly acclaimed manual of freestyle shamanism, Suitable for all those inspired by such figures as Austin Spare and Aleister Crowley, and who feel the imperative to develop one's own unique magick way. Visual Magick aims to build vision, imagination, and creative magick. It shows how magicians, witches, artists and therapists can improve visionary abilities, enhance imagination, activate the inner senses, and discover new modes of Trance awareness. The emphasis is on direct experience and the reader is asked to think, act, do, and enjoy as s/he wills.

**Visit our website: www.mandrake.uk.net
or call for a catalogue on +44 (0)1865 243671
email mandrake@mandrake.uk.net
write to: PO Box 250, Oxford, OX1 1AP (UK)**

www.ingramcontent.com/pod-product-compliance
Lightning Source LLC
LaVergne TN
LVHW010338260326
834688LV00036B/763